Praise for
Holistic Cancer Medicine

"Dr. Saupe's comprehensive new book shows that there is so much a person can do to treat and prevent cancer in addition to conventional medicine. If you want to gain a thorough understanding of cancer cells and the immune system, I highly recommend *Holistic Cancer Medicine*."

—KELLY A. TURNER, PhD, *New York Times* bestselling author of *Radical Hope* and *Radical Remission*

"We need a new path forward in the realm of cancer; not only for the way we think about the formation of this devastating process but also in its treatment. Dr. Henning Saupe's new book accomplishes both of those things by reworking the very foundation of cancer science, making this a 'must read' for anyone serious about understanding how cancer begins and what we can do about it."

—DR. CHRIS CHLEBOWSKI, author of *The Virus and the Host*

"Dr. Saupe is one of the few medical professionals who truly understands the meaning of 'holistic' in the context of treating cancer. In *Holistic Cancer Medicine*, Dr. Saupe not only covers specific treatment strategies that can be key to recovery and healing, he also addresses the limitations of certain treatment and diagnostic approaches, and how to incorporate them effectively. Dr. Saupe tackles delicate and complex discussions in a highly approachable, humble, and practical way without being overwhelming or dogmatic, and the scientific rationale he offers will leave you in awe of both the simplicity and complexity of the human body—and what it truly means to heal and recover."

—PATRICIA DALY, coauthor of *The Ketogenic Kitchen*

Holistic Cancer Medicine

Holistic Cancer Medicine

Integrative Strategies
for a New Approach to
Health and Healing

Henning Saupe, MD

Chelsea Green Publishing
White River Junction, Vermont
London, UK

Originally published in Germany by VAK Verlags GmbH, Eschbachstraße 5, 79199 Kirchzarten, Germany, www.vakverlag.de, in 2021 as *Krebs verstehen und ganzheitlich behandeln*.

This edition published by Chelsea Green Publishing, 2022.

Note: The purpose of this book is to provide information about health care possibilities. Those who use it do so at their own risk. The author and the publisher do not intend to make diagnoses or give recommendations for therapy. The procedures described here are not intended as a substitute for professional medical treatment for cancer or other serious health conditions.

Project Manager: Patricia Stone
Project Editor: Brianne Goodspeed
Copy Editor: Deborah Heimann
Proofreader: Nancy A. Crompton
Indexer: Shana Milkie
Designer: Melissa Jacobson

Printed in Canada.
First printing October 2022.
10 9 8 7 6 5 4 3 2 1   22 23 24 25 26

ISBN 978-1-64502-155-1 (paperback) | ISBN 978-1-64502-156-8 (ebook) | ISBN 978-1-64502-157-5 (audio book)

Library of Congress Cataloging-in-Publication Data is available upon request.

Chelsea Green Publishing
85 North Main Street, Suite 120
White River Junction, Vermont USA

Somerset House
London, UK

www.chelseagreen.com

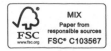

For Emanuel, David, and Fredrik, my sons

Contents

Prologue   *xi*

Introduction. The Holistic Principle   1

1 Who Suffers from Cancer and
Who Profits from This Suffering   15

2 How the Light Shines   23

3 The Holistic Model of the
Twelve Vital Fields   30

4 Balance: Everything in Flux   155

5 Complementary Oncology   159

6 Cancer Therapies: Outside the Box   178

Epilogue. Cancer and a Good Life
Are Not Mutually Exclusive   236

Acknowledgments   239
Notes   241
References   242
Index   255

Prologue

As human beings, we are constantly exposed to influences that can make us healthy or ill. From conception and birth, and throughout life until our last breath, life is in a constant state of flux, building up and breaking down the substances that make up the human body and its organism. Nothing in us ever stands still.

The infinitely nuanced network of forces that holds our body together for as long as it serves us in our life is referred to in traditional Eastern medical teachings as *chi* (Chinese), *qi* (Japanese), or *prana* (Sanskrit, ancient Indian), and in anthroposophical medicine, which was developed in the 1920s, it is understood as the interaction of "life force body," "soul body," and "I-organization."

We simply call it *vital force*, and naturopathy speaks of the self-healing powers that have their origin in this vital force.

Naturopathy's approach is to restoratively influence this field of forces and to restore the self-regulation of the immune system, to reorganize the coherence of the forces of the psyche (soul) and soma (body), thus eliminating life's constantly occurring obstacles that lead to ailments and diseases, and to always make new life possible.

———

Cancer is the consequence of a disturbance of these highly complex interrelationships, a disturbance of the vital forces of the human being. This disturbance is what this book is about. The more we understand about it, the better we can protect ourselves from cancer by living a health-conscious life. The more we know about what might help to induce cancer, the better we can deal with it, sometimes cure it, or at least bring it under control and integrate it into our lives, so that we can then live with confidence and in a (more) conscious way.

———

Follow me on a journey through the laws and phenomena of health and illness! Learn to understand more and more how everything we do or refrain from doing, feel or repress, ingest or have a deficiency of, influences our risk of getting cancer or recovering from it, so that from now on you can live in a way that is good for you, and can do more of what is really important and valuable to you.

Introduction

The Holistic Principle

I have based this book on the holistic principle. The ancient Greek term *hólos* means "whole," and *hólon* means "the being that is part of a whole." My conviction and experience is that everything is connected to everything else and that nothing can be or be considered as a single, detached part independent of other parts or influences.

We can still consider an individual cell as a whole, but it is also part of a larger whole, for example the organ. We can also consider the organ as a whole, but it, too, is part of a larger whole, namely the body, and so on. In both directions, getting smaller and getting larger, we can imagine this hierarchy of *hólons* and a world whose parts can be considered individually, but also relate to one another in a larger context.

Thus, in terms of the human organism, the holistic principle means that each part is in mutual exchange with a larger whole. The system of the human organism reacts as a whole and is not to be understood solely as the sum of its components: Each cell reacts to influences from the whole organism, and the whole organism reacts to the influences from each cell. The human body is thus also like a hologram, in which each part reflects the whole and the properties of the parts can be found in the whole.

This insight, that the design principle of the human being is reflected in the universe, has been described by numerous philosophers over the centuries as the correlation between the microcosm (the human being) and the macrocosm (the world).

The texts of the *Tabula Smaragdina* (Emerald Tablet) are said to trace back to Hermes Trismegistos, who was supposedly a fusion of the Greek god

Hermes and the Egyptian god Thoth and who was said to have actually lived. They are the philosophical basis of hermeticism, which lies at the heart of the collected writings of the *Corpus Hermeticum*, which was composed by a group of Neoplatonists in Greece in the first to third century AD, and was rediscovered during the Renaissance in the fifteenth century by Cosimo di Medici and translated into Latin.

The concept of this correlation is also reflected there: "As above, so below; as within, so without; as the mind, so the body" was the philosophical guiding principle of ancient natural science and of medicine as an art of healing, which emerged slowly over the centuries.

From Greek antiquity until the middle of the nineteenth century, the understanding of the hermetic laws sufficed with the correlation of the large world (macrocosm / universe) and the small world (microcosm / human being).

The relationships in the universe correspond to this view, according to which, in the individual, the external conditions are reflected in human beings and vice versa. Changes in the microcosmic sphere consequently also have an effect on the totality.

This philosophical school also decisively shaped the thinking and actions of the greatest physician of antiquity: Hippocrates of Kos, the founder of modern medicine and humoral pathology. He developed the Theory of the Four Humors, the essence of which is that health is based on a balance (Greek *krasis*, Latin *humores*), and illness on an imbalance (Greek *dyskrasis*) of the inner forces.

The four forces that should be balanced were first referred to as the "Four Elements" doctrine by Empedocles (a pre-Socratic philosopher who was born around 495 BC in Sicily and died around 435 BC, presumably in the Peloponnese). The properties of fire, water, air, and earth corresponded to the humors blood, phlegm, yellow bile, and black bile in the human being.

In ancient times, however, these terms were to be understood as relating to a process rather than anything biochemically material. The important aspect for us here is that health was understood as the balance of forces.

There is a late-medieval depiction of this principle of forces, in which the human being finds themselves, in an image from the book of hours *Les Très Riches Heures du Duc de Berry*.

This masterpiece of book illumination is the most famous illustrated manuscript of the fifteenth century and was painted by the Limbourg brothers for their master Johann von Berry. The core is formed by the elaborately designed and detailed calendar pages. It illustrates important stories from the Bible, including all annual celebrations, and it shows, as a special feature, the depiction of *l'homme anatomique*, the anatomical man, as he is integrated into the forces of the cosmos (see figure 1 in the color insert).

Amid four groups of zodiac signs that are each assigned one of the four elements (fire, water, air, and earth), an organ, a temperament, a cardinal direction, and the qualities damp, dry, warm, and cold, the human being stands as a female-male twofold being.

This image expresses the principle of the analogy of hermeticism like no other—the duality of all being—and should serve here as an example of pictorially capturing the concept of a comprehensive force field from which illness or health arises. It also clearly shows that this knowledge has a long philosophical prehistory.

The medical-philosophical doctrine of the Hippocratic theory of the humors was set out for the last time in modern times in 1848 by the Austrian pathologist and philosopher Karl von Rokitansky (1804–1878) in his scientific textbook, *General Pathological Anatomy*.

The pathologist Rudolf Virchow from Berlin (1821–1902) established the reductionist theory of disease only a few years later in his book *Cellular Pathology*, published in 1858, and became world-famous due to its dissemination. The consequences and effects of Virchow's reductionism are still the predominant philosophical guideline of Western medicine today. "Diseases arise from diseased cells" was the new dogma from which the reductionist-materialist approach to medicine developed and is still favored today by so-called conventional medicine.

Using the microscope, it was possible to see more and more details, which were interpreted as the causes of diseases. It was no longer the person who was ill, it was their cells. And soon it was no longer just the cells, but parts of the cells—receptors on the surface of the cell membrane, genes (i.e., DNA segments inside the nucleus or individual molecules)—that were held responsible for the development of the diseases. The understanding of the whole fell apart in favor of a vast multitude of individual phenomena.

For more than two thousand years prior to this, disease and health were understood as dynamic processes between the imbalance and balance of forces.

More recently, Karl H. Pribram (1919–2015), an Austrian-American neuroscientist, together with the quantum physicist David Bohm (1917–1992), developed a "holonomic brain model" in the 1960s.

In this model, Pribram attributed a "field character" to the brain and argued that the brain should be understood as a whole and not as individual neurons that make it up: "Our brain is a hologram which interprets a holographic universe" is one of his well-known quotes.

The challenge of our time therefore lies in integrating the newly acquired findings and the enormous (biochemical) knowledge into a larger whole and merging individual pieces of the mosaic, which on their own are "complete" and "functional" little stones in color and form, with others to form a picture, which in turn forms a larger whole.

A processual understanding of illness and health can still be found today in the Ayurvedic act of healing, which originated in India and has been practiced and scientifically taught there for over 2,500 years. It is based on a conception of the human being in which the unity of body, mind, and soul is in constant interaction with the environment. Here, health is synonymous with the balance of metabolism, digestion, body tissues, and excretions and is dependent on the inner well-being of the consciousness, mind, and senses, while the body goes through a multitude of complex metabolic processes every second.

Traditional Chinese Medicine (TCM), which was developed in China about two thousand years ago and is taught scientifically today, also demonstrates this balance of forces with the balance of yin and yang.

In the Indian and Chinese arts of healing and medicine and the associated conception of the human being, the life force is still an established concept and part of both the philosophy and the practice. The Chinese term for life force is *chi*, the Indian is *prana*, and the Greek is *bios*. The vitalists of the nineteenth century, tracing back to Aristotle, called it *vis vitalis* (Latin for "life force").

Today, we have become accustomed to the fact that the term *life* is understood either not at all or only abstractly, and that we have no clear definition for *life* and no longer have an exact understanding of it.

In the study of medicine in our western latitudes and time, the term *life* is practically no longer used; it is neither studied nor taught. This is also why we have no reasonable definition of *health* in conventional medicine. The "absence of disease," which is the World Health Organization (WHO)'s valid definition of *health*, is only a deferral of the problem, not a solution.

According to the WHO, human health is "a state of complete physical, mental and social well-being," and not just the absence of disease or infirmity.

Complexity and Unambiguity

Today we know that more than one hundred thousand biochemical reactions take place every second in each of our approximately one hundred trillion body cells. From these figures alone, it is clear that we cannot begin to understand or predict what controls the living cell and exactly how it will behave. An astonishing observation, a careful description is still the scientist's noble way of approaching the immeasurably complex living cell and the even more complex human organism.

There is still a long way to go before we have a precise understanding of all the details, a grasp of the concrete connections between cause and effect, and a prediction of the complete cellular behavior.

It seems rather as if the number of possible reactions of a cell goes to infinity, similar to the number of all possible chess games, estimated to be 10^{100}, which is very close to infinity (e.g., 10^{100} exceeds the number of electrons in the known, visible universe).

These numerical examples of the complexity of biochemical processes in the human organism show that there cannot be a simple or one answer to the problem of cancer. The number of factors that influence cancer is very high and the number of possible combinations of these is even higher.

The above-mentioned examples should help us to not fall into the trap of wanting to find the one factor that triggers cancer and the one therapy that cures it.

Rather, our understanding of the multifactorial etiology (history of development) of the various cancers results in a multitude of different treatment options. It is indeed a great task to find and apply the treatments that are best for the individual case, but it is also the only sensible way.

The therapy of an individual person should therefore consist of typical treatments that are useful and effective for most people with the disease—including, for example, the reduction of inflammation and stress—as well as those adapted to the individual factors of each person, which include, for example, the use of individually adapted amounts of nutritional supplements, lesion and interference field recovery (tooth root infections, chronically inflamed throat and tonsils, etc.), and specific lifestyle changes.

Here, it is important to always keep an eye on the big picture and to remedy the weak points first. Step by step, the treatment should be guided by these questions: "What can be changed most quickly with the least effort?" and "What causes the most damage?"

If your work or family environment is a major stress factor in your life, this should be changed before, for example, any amalgam fillings in the teeth are removed. When materials such as gold, amalgam, and other metal alloys are found in the tooth region, which then trigger chemical reactions via the saliva, like a battery, and afflict the organism with the corresponding toxins, the general advice is to replace amalgam fillings with metal-free materials, if possible. This advice is correct in principle, but must be compared with the other therapy elements against the background of their importance. Even if these fillings are not conducive to health, they play a rather subordinate role in the overall process in this example. Priorities should be sensibly assessed in the overall treatment, and treatment options should be weighed.

Here, the insight of Lofti Zadeh (1921–2017), an American mathematician, computer scientist, electrical engineer, and professor emeritus of computer science, can also help us; this is because there will never be exact or mathematical certainty in such complex systems, and a certain uncertainty will always remain.

Zadeh coined the term *fuzzy logic* in 1965 and developed a new method of dealing with fuzzy information. *Fuzzy* means blurry, indistinct, or unclear. His term does not refer to any specific mathematic logic, as one might think, but rather a theory—the theory of *fuzzy sets*.

Although he had a background in mathematics and computer science, Zadeh was convinced early on that his theory would be applied in the field of medical diagnosis, and believed that we needed to change our traditional approaches to the analysis of biological systems in a fundamental way, as the complexity of such biological systems was too multifaceted to be calculated with monocausal parameters. He said: "To the extent that the complexity of a system increases, precise statements lose their meaning and meaningful statements lose their precision."

In science or computer programming, only two values were used until this point: true or false, on or off, 0 or 1. There were no intermediate values or grey areas. We are used to dividing the world into a black-and-white grid, even though this *either–or* does not correspond to our actual experience. We thereby reduce the world to two values and behave as if there were no transition between these extremes.

The binary representation makes mathematics and computer processing (more) manageable. Yet the result obtained in this way can—sometimes more, sometimes less—be a fallacy. Our age of information is indeed based on this digital way of thinking and working, but it cannot sufficiently calculate or classify complex biological systems such as our life.

Since antiquity, philosophy, among other things, has been dealing with the question of fuzzy sets, for example, in the form of the famous sorites paradox and the question: "At what point does a collection of sand grains become a heap?"

How many or how few hairs on your head do you have to have to be bald, or how many cancerous cells need to be present in the body to make a person ill? It is very difficult to draw a line here, but by simplifying we often succumb to a misjudgment.

Even if correlations are not immediately obvious, this does not mean that they do not exist. Life is multifactorial and therefore sometimes feels unpredictable, erratic, and chaotic. Just like the rest of life, it is the same in medicine: The lack of evidence of a correlation is not evidence that there is no correlation. Thus the danger is that we deny correlations where we don't see any ostensible ones. However, this approach does not do justice to a holistic (world) view.

A study carried out in 2017 by the geneticist and tumor researcher Bert Vogelstein and his colleague, the mathematician and statistician Cristian Tomasetti from the Johns Hopkins University in Baltimore, provides a provocative answer to the question of cancer development in the journal *Science*: In two out of three cases, the tumor formation was due to pure chance, to "typing errors" in copying the genetic information before cell division. According to this study, cancer is pure coincidence and simply "bad luck," a fateful event that is not caused in any way by the sufferers. Thus, the two researchers strike the general tone of Western conventional medicine.

On the one hand, the result of this study may be a relief for some people and can be particularly relieving regarding the questions "Why me?" and "What did I do wrong?," which presumably almost all cancer patients ask. However, this view absolves us of any responsibility we have toward ourselves and our bodies that influences our lifestyles. According to this view, it would make no difference what and how we eat, whether we exercise and get enough sleep, whether we seek and find meaning in life, whether we surround ourselves with people and animals who are good for us, whether we live by certain values and impart them, and whether we continue to develop ourselves. Everything we do and think would therefore not matter. Everything would effectively be bad luck and sheer coincidence.

However, we advocate taking responsibility for ourselves and thereby achieving a certain degree of co-determination and self-determination in our lives. Even if the interplay of many disease-promoting factors remains unrecognized or cannot be deciphered down to the last detail, we are not just helplessly at the mercy of bad luck or chance.

With the holistic model of the twelve vital fields, we assume that the development of cancer is a highly complex, multifactorial occurrence, but that we can positively influence this occurrence very well by dealing with the twelve vital fields and can change it significantly. By paying attention to the different fields and taking responsibility for ourselves mentally and physically, we are not just at the mercy of fate, but can approach cancer (or any kind of illness) not only differently, but also actively. Hippocrates was of the opinion that most diseases are caused by lifestyle and are not sent by the gods. The holistic view and method of treatment can accordingly lead to useful and successful therapy as a whole.

Coherence and Health

The human organism is seen in this book not only holistically, but as being influenced by twelve different principles. The special thing about these principles—which can be seen as risk factors in the case of cancer—is that they are not material. They influence the composition and behavior of matter, but are themselves immaterial. They are ultimately forces that constantly act on the living cells and organs of our bodies and are connected to one another

The Twelve Vital Fields

1. Detoxification
2. Nutrition
3. Water
4. Oxygen
5. Gut health
6. Stress management
7. Blood sugar regulation
8. Immunity
9. Mitochondrial health
10. Acid-base balance
11. Infection control
12. Inflammation control

as twelve fields and are in constant exchange like the colors of sunlight. To divide them into twelve nuances is like looking at a prism that breaks down the white sunlight into its colored components.

Life itself is hidden behind the twelve factors presented here.

The objective of this book is to help those affected by cancer to be able to formulate an active, vibrant concept of life for themselves again. A dynamic understanding of life is presented and explained here, a principle that is not only material but also spiritual and that underlies the biochemical processes of the organism and organizes and shapes them in the sense of a force field.

The twelve factors discussed here can be understood like twelve instruments of an orchestra. The conductor of an orchestra is the human being themselves, determined by inherited dispositions (genes—they cannot be influenced) and epigenetic structures (they can be influenced by one's own behavior and the environment). The "sound of music" is the biography of the human being. In this image, out-of-tune instruments—which play incoherently, disjointedly and each for themselves—lead to distortion of the music, which is in our case to diseases.

The therapy is thus the tuning of the instruments, the vitalizing of the twelve factors and making them coherent with one another, into an order, a correlation, and an interconnected relationship.

By analogy with the field concept commonly used in physics—which, for example, arranges the structure of iron filings on a sheet of paper as a magnetic field as soon as the force field of a magnet acts underneath the paper—the totality of the effective (and in the best case regulative) influencing factors is also referred to as a *field* in this book.

The arrangement of the iron filings comes from the force field of the magnet, not from the iron filings themselves. In our opinion, the "disease cancer" does not come from the diseased cells, but rather is caused by the manifold forces, the biochemical processes around them that the cells follow like the iron filings follow the magnetic field.

When cancer presents itself as a disease, it is not the cancer cell itself that has a *problem*, but rather the human being, whose physical—as well as mental-spiritual—existence is threatened and endangered to the highest degree.

According to the understanding on which this book is based, the human being has an extremely complex and multilayered essence. The word *essence*, which also means the "special part" or "characterizing part," points to a meaning, to something spiritual. This spiritual thing uses something physical in order to be able to express itself and evolve. The essence of the human being is not only multilayered, but also expresses itself on numerous levels. A classical approach, which gets somewhat closer to the elusive concept of the human being, classifies it into *body* and *soul*.

A more refined classification distinguishes the soul and spirit as two different areas. The body can in turn be classified as a mineral or physical body and a biochemical body. As long as it is in a state of health, its main feature is to maintain the pulsating balance between decomposition and construction. This state is also referred to with the ancient Greek term *homeostasis*, which means "equilibrium" and also describes this balanced state of a dynamic system maintained by internal regulatory processes.

The physical body separates itself from the biochemical body in this way by appearing as a solid structure. The biochemical body, on the other hand, is constantly changing and flows, pulsates, breathes, oscillates back and forth, contracts, expands, grows, and transforms.

What the soul is has a different meaning depending on mythical, religious, philosophical, or psychological traditions and teachings. According to many people's understanding today, it is the place or space, belonging to the physical body, that perceives emotions and receives impressions. The soul is conceived of as something inner and is the personality trait of a human being. Originating from the ancient Greek, *soul* means "psyche." When we speak of psychological health, we mean the spiritual-mental state, without wanting to distinguish it too much for our observations here.

So while we are somewhat cautious defining what the soul is, we can say with certainty that it—whatever it is—reacts. And the soul interacts to the highest degree with the biochemical organism.

In medicine today, we assume that physis and psyche, that is, body and mind or soul, are dependent on each other and influence each other.

Psychoimmunology (also called psychoneuroimmunology, or PNI for short) and, particularly for our consideration, psycho-oncology or psycho-social oncology are important, as well as the science of the interactions of these different planes of the human essence.

Here, we are not just talking about the interactions between the psyche, nervous system, and immune system, but specifically about the psychological and social conditions, consequences, and accompanying effects of cancer.

If we follow these interactions, they lead us to the Israeli-American medical sociologist Aaron Antonovsky (1923–1994), who coined the term *salutogenesis* in the 1980s, which translates from Latin as "becoming healthy."

In his salutogenesis model, the concept of coherence (from the Latin *cohaehere*, meaning "interrelated" or "connected") plays a central role: Antonovsky also understood the development and preservation of health as an active process with dynamic interactions and not as a passive state.

He placed this sense of coherence at the center of the development of health, which describes a person's ability to use the resources available to them in order to stay healthy. Antonovsky found the influencing factors of understanding, feasibility, and meaningfulness particularly important.

Similar to his salutogenesis model, in which a meaningful and coherent interplay of different influencing factors is significant, this book shows how a coherent intertwining of the twelve factors engenders good health, whereas a lack of coherence promotes disease and ultimately cancer.

But what is coherence in a healthy state? And what does coherence mean in the context of illness, when we are physically as well as psychologically weakened or ailing? What becomes disordered in the ill state of the human being? What does this coherence consist of and what effect does it have on the human being?

The coherence, or the interplay of the different levels, divided into the physical body, the chemical processes in the body, and mental-spiritual matters, occurs on very different levels. If it is imbalanced, the lack of coherence is evident in the area of the physical (body) as a deforming-tumor formation (i.e., proliferation and formation of substance in the wrong place) and is seen in pathologically increased intensity.

In the field of biochemical processes, the absence of coherence leads to chronic inflammation, immunological aberration, local hyperacidity, local oxygen deficiency, or local toxic load.

In the area of psychological sensation or experience, its absence manifests itself as a loss of meaningful connections in thinking, feeling, and wanting, as well as being anxious and deficient.

In the specific field of the mind, the lack of coherence manifests itself through the loss of the meaningful, proportional, and therefore healthy relationship between self-perception and external perception. Here, the weighing up and realization of one's own needs, which are either in line with the needs of the environment or in opposition to them, becomes a partially insurmountable obstacle.

Without consciously perceiving it, there is a sufficiently high coherence between these different levels of the human being as long as they are healthy. This coherence maintains the shape of the body, regulates its energetic needs, which are expressed in the transformation of biochemical activities, allows us to react appropriately, and maintains the balance in the relationship between the self and the environment.

In his work "Reflexive Social Psychology," the social psychologist Heiner Keupp (1943–) described coherence as a feeling and called it "the sense of coherence." He divided it into three areas:

Coherence is the feeling that there is a correlation and sense in life, that life is not subject to an uninfluenceable fate. The sense of coherence describes a mental attitude: to me, my world appears understandable, harmonious, orderly; I can even see the problems and burdens that I experience in a larger context (comprehensibility).

Life presents me with tasks that I can solve. I have resources that I can mobilize to master my life, my current problems (manageability). Every effort makes sense for the way I lead my life. There are goals and projects that are worth committing myself to (meaningfulness). The state of demoralization forms the antithesis of the sense of coherence.

It seems, however, that the sense of comprehensibility, manageability, and meaningfulness—in short, the sense of coherence—is weakened, or in some cases even completely undermined, by illness.

In fact, even when we are suffering from a flu-like infection, it is difficult to have a sunny disposition, to be in a positive and energetic mood and to look into the future optimistically: When we are ill, we feel mentally as well as physically frail, more emotionally vulnerable, less energetic (which is of course also due to our purely physical condition) and less able to make decisions, no longer able to cope with the demands of our fellow human beings, our own, and those of daily life. We feel overwhelmed, much smaller, and more defenseless. The range of feelings that accompany illness can manifest themselves distinctly in each person; some people retreat particularly quietly and try to manage everything themselves, while others may become weepy, clingy, whiny, or reproachful.

The demoralization that comes with illness can look different depending on your age. But in the case of a flu-like infection, a cold, an uncomplicated bone fracture, dental treatment, and so forth, it is a manageable and conceivable period in our lives that we learn to deal with as we grow older, and we know how to assess it as adults.

Life-threatening diseases such as cancer, on the other hand, have much more power over our equilibrium and have a very different impact on unhinging our coherence. There are no simple answers to the questions "Why me?" and "What did I do wrong?" Feelings of guilt lead to further mental stress and thus also to an additional weakening of the entire system, but not to a solution.

Because illness is partly caused by a loss of coherence, and a lack of coherence furthermore negatively influences the organism, a solution to the problem and thus the support of health can be achieved only through a change of direction. It must also work the other way around, that coherence is established and solidified when we reflect on what is good for us, on how we want to live, how we want to treat other living beings, what we need and what we should avoid, what we want to demand but also what we should refuse, what we desire, and what we can do. Small steps in the realm of the feasible are particularly important and for most of us, even in good health, part of our daily routine.

Living with cancer means being attentive, consciously shaping our everyday life, and developing a high degree of observation for small changes in the body. Cancer in the metastasized stage remains a permanent challenge: Only holistic treatment and aftercare can regulate or repress the progression of cancer.

Chapter One

Who Suffers from Cancer and Who Profits from This Suffering

1.1 Cancer on the Rise

In all modern civilizations, cancer is one of the greatest challenges for people who may be concerned about their lives and their health. There are approximately five hundred different diseases that the layperson refers to with the collective term *cancer*, and cases continue to be on the rise in Western civilizations and are on their way to overtaking cardiovascular diseases, such as heart attacks and strokes, as the leading cause of death. In Canada, it has already reached this point: Cancer is the number one cause of death there.

The trend in all developed industrial nations of our modern world is dramatic: Every year, there are about 2 percent more cancer diagnoses than in the previous year, and by 2040, statistically one in two adults will get cancer if we do not stop this development and learn to fundamentally strengthen our health.

Before we use this book to delve further into the interplay between life forces and the influences that cause disease, it is important to create a picture of the current state of cancer and how it occurs in the world.

In order for us to better understand what the landscape of oncology departments in our hospitals looks like, what range of treatment methods are practiced there and why oncology research in our universities is the way it is (and does not follow what, for example, this book describes, reveals, and recommends), it is interesting to look at the scientific and economic aspects of cancer.

Facts and Figures

The information service of the German Cancer Research Center published the following disease rates on its website in 2020: "In 2016, about 492,000 people were newly diagnosed with cancer in Germany. For 2020, an increase to more than 500,000 new cases of cancer is predicted. If you compare these figures with the situation in 1970, the number of cancer sufferers has almost doubled. There are various reasons for this: the increase in life expectancy and the decline in other diseases that used to be life-threatening play a role. Almost all types of cancer occur much more frequently in older people than in younger people."

In 2017, 226,680 people died of cancer in Germany. It is estimated that in Germany—with a population of about 83 million people—there are approximately 1.67 million cancer patients who were diagnosed with cancer no more than five years ago. Overall, more than half of all cancer patients today are still alive five years after their diagnosis. This means that the other half of people with cancer do not survive these five years. These figures are very different for the various types of cancer, which we cannot go into in detail in this book. Transnationally, the four most common cancers are breast cancer, lung cancer, colorectal cancer, and prostate cancer. When cancer is discussed in this book, we usually refer to the commonplace and most frequently occurring types of cancer. The types of blood cancer (e.g., leukemia) are specific diseases, which require specific representation. Some general aspects of leukemia are dealt with in this book, but not the specific ones, as they would go beyond the scope of this book.

In an international comparison of countries, there are very big differences in terms of the number of new cancer cases per year. This comparison shows a clear picture: The Western industrialized nations (Western Europe, North America, Australia, and New Zealand) are at the top of the table, by a large margin in comparison to the other countries, with over 253 and up to 450 new cases of cancer per 100,000 inhabitants per year. India and the African and Arabic countries close to the equator have the lowest number of new cases, namely under 106 per 100,000 people per year. These differences seem to correlate less to genetic factors than to lifestyle factors. What is particularly striking is that Japanese women have a much lower risk of breast cancer (approximately 53 new cases per 100,000 inhabitants per year) than European, Australian, or American women do (about 85–94 new cases per 100,000 inhabitants per year). If Japanese women move to one of the countries with a high incidence of cancer, their risk will become the same as that of their new country of residence after a few years! This means that the cause of their higher risk of cancer is not due to their genes, but is influenced by lifestyle and environmental factors. Chinese men have just under one-tenth of the incidence of prostate cancer (about 9 new cases per 100,000 inhabitants per year) in comparison to men in Western civilizations (about 75–85 new cases per 100,000 inhabitants per year). So the burning question is: Why does our Western lifestyle promote cancer to such a high extent?

1.2 Cancer and the Associated Industry . . . a Blessing for Humanity or "Big Business"?

With this enormous spread throughout the whole industrialized world and its accompanying significance for the health of modern man, it is perhaps not surprising that an entire industry and a research world supporting it have been formed. Alongside the goal of being able to better treat cancer, economic interests are—and sometimes we would like to say, *unfortunately*—also pursued. The interdependence of research institutes and the pharmaceutical industry is a complex subject that already fills many books and that we will only touch on here.

For the basic understanding of this reading, it is important to mention that a book such as this one is considered as *alternative*. Notwithstanding that it is based on biological facts and reflects the latest knowledge in various scientific fields, it cannot be considered as a popular general representative of the prevailing doctrine that is applied in the oncology clinics in our Western, industrialized countries.

But what actually is the *doctrine* represented so uniformly in universities and the generally accepted *conventional medicine*, and how does this often one-sided view of disease come about?

For the field of oncology, the answer is this: The conventional medical doctrine is that which has been "sufficiently" scientifically researched at the respective point in time and which is proven by evidence-based studies.

Simplified, one could also say that it is the doctrine that academic teachers and professors of Western-oriented universities define as the *correct* one. This is a circular argument, which is akin to a self-contained system that sets its own rules and acts in accordance with them, while much else is dismissed as unscientific.

The first thing that stands out is a significant error in thinking: What has not been proven with evidence-based studies should not, by implication, be regarded as wrong per se. It is just not proven by the mainstream-influenced (or funded) science and its standards.

EXAMPLE

The soothing effect of a hot water bottle on the stomach of a patient with menstrual pain has not been proven to be effective in any study. However, this does not make it false, ineffective, or unscientific. It is part of empirical medicine and is a frequently applied practice. This example may seem banal, but it hits the nail on the head.

––––––––

Only that which is backed up by large controlled randomized studies is included in the guidelines for standard oncological treatments. In most Western countries, this is not only a *recommendation*, but is a requirement that tolerates no exceptions. In France or Sweden, for example, only procedures or drugs that have been "backed up" by large controlled randomized studies are used. Unfortunately, this means that a lot remains unnoticed and ultimately cannot benefit patients. In German-speaking and some Asian countries, the regulations are a little more relaxed, and the above-mentioned empirical medicine may also be used.

A study is randomized if it consists of two groups, the participants of which are randomly selected. One group gets the drug to be studied, the other gets the usual standard. It is placebo-controlled if the control group is given an ineffective pseudo-drug (from Latin *placere*, which roughly means *to please*, i.e., to *give the appearance* of being a drug).

It is best if a study of this kind is planned in advance (prospective) and is carried out in several places at the same time (multicentered). The expenditure of such studies can only be guessed at. The costs amount to seven- to eight-figure sums. Before a new anticancer drug is freely available, it has to undergo four phases of clinical trials with the means just described. Before it is introduced to the market or sold at all, it costs the company in question around five billion euros. This figure alone makes it clear why anticancer remedies such as high-dosage vitamin C, mistletoe extracts, or curcumin do not stand a chance of being included in the guidelines for recommended (and thus also health-insurance-financed) cancer treatments in the foreseeable future: High-dosage vitamin C, mistletoe, and curcuma extract are very inexpensive to procure and produce compared to other medicines, which unfortunately now means that such remedies have a reputation of not being "as effective" as expensive medications, and their use is unlikely to generate the money that pharmaceutical companies want to develop their drugs and to test whether they are effective or not and to what extent.

The cost of cancer treatment has increased a hundredfold in the last fifty-five years! In 1965, an average of around one hundred US dollars a month was spent per cancer patient; today it's about ten thousand US dollars.

Unfortunately, many of the expensive anticancer drugs available today do not work at all, or work much less than we would like.

The English cancer researcher, professor, and oncologist Charles Swanton summarized the sobering figures in an article he published in the *Royal Society of Medicine* journal in 2018: "If we take the last twelve years and look at the seventy-one new anticancer remedies accepted by the *Food and Drug Administration* between 2002 and 2014, 23 of these drugs have shown no survival benefit at all. Overall, the average improvement in survival was 2.1 months. This was similar to the case with drugs approved in Europe. Forty-eight drugs were approved for sixty-eight different indications (areas of application). In forty-one of these sixty-eight areas of application, there was no improvement in survival at all. I would argue that the costs are not in proportion to the advantages, something that needs to be addressed immediately."

In addition, there is a completely different, less praiseworthy aspect of modern connections between research, the pharmaceutical industry, and attending physicians, namely fraud.

The Danish university professor Peter Christian Gøtzsche, the cofounder and director of the renowned Cochrane Institute in Copenhagen until 2018, exposed and criticized the machinations of the power of the pharmaceutical industry, which reaches into political structures, in his courageous book *Deadly Medicines and Organised Crime: How Big Pharma Has Corrupted Healthcare*.

There is a lot of money at stake. In 2015, it was estimated that over 107 billion US dollars was spent on anticancer drugs worldwide, and sales are expected to reach 150 billion US dollars by 2020. Currently, 511 different pharmaceutical companies have 581 potential anticancer drugs in mid-stage testing, with the hope of some of them getting approved. A single drug can generate a turnover of 4 billion US dollars a year, with a profit margin of about 70 percent! A single treatment with a series of infusions of a new drug can cost well over a million US dollars.

In modern oncology, new drugs that intervene in the immune system in a very specific way are becoming more and more popular. Unfortunately, they also have many side effects. A current example are the checkpoint inhibitors. They block a signaling module that is found on almost all healthy cells and some cancer cells and signals to the immune system not to attack them. By *masking* these programmed cell death-1 receptors (PD-1 receptors), the inhibition of cancer cells attacking the immune system is switched off. According to a report from 2020, two such drugs, which have been on the market for several years, are valued at 2.637 billion euros and account for 6.6 percent of the total cost of drugs from a whole year of statutory health insurance funds.

At the time this book was written, the drug therapy with the highest cost was CAR T-cell therapy, in which special white blood cells are taken from the blood of the person being treated and then modified in the laboratory to then be injected back into the patient. A single injection of this substance, which is produced individually for each patient, cost 475,000 US dollars (approximately 435,000 euros) when launched in the United States.

Usually, three such injections are given to a person to be treated in a treatment attempt. In comparison, the price of a kilogram of vitamin C for consumers is less than twenty euros. There is no money to be made here. This comparison is not meant to claim that vitamin C is as strong as a modern immunotherapy drug, nor does it have strong side effects, which, for the group of the above-mentioned checkpoint inhibitors, occur in up to 89 percent of those treated, as shown in the *Deutsches Ärzteblatt* in 2019. The comparison is intended only to show the vast differences in the costs of anticancer drugs.

In addition, those with health insurance in Germany have to pay for the cost of, for example, high-dosage vitamin C or vitamin D, which is extremely effective for cancer prevention and treatment, themselves, because the guidelines do not allow for treatment with these vitamins. However, the more you go into this matter, the better you understand how we have created a self-contained system that dominates all of medicine, but especially oncology. In no other field of medicine is so much money turned over for drugs.

1.3 The Self-Contained System of Medical Research

"Human life is deplorable, because the unbearable greed for money permeates it through and through like an icy breath. May all doctors stand together against it with the will of curing a disease completely."[1]

Our medical system consists of the self-contained cycle, because university research—ideally independent—is largely financed or supported by the industry. Only drugs that promise correspondingly high profits are researched and investigated in large clinical trials. Drugs that are not expected to generate a large profit are not investigated in the first place.

Guidelines are set out by professors who have made their careers with the help of studies financed by third-party funds. Unfortunately, the saying "He who pays the piper, calls the tune" is all too often true, and so the guidelines do not include any treatment measures or drugs that have not been investigated in large and cost-intensive trials. Health insurance companies almost always pay only for treatments that are proposed in the guidelines, and refuse to reimburse treatments that do not conform to these guidelines.

So if, while reading this book, the question arises as to why this content has not found its way into oncological clinics and their treatment methods, the facts presented here can provide an answer.

Possible Escape from Money-Based Medicine

The public health system—consisting of universities, researchers, health insurers, and doctors—largely ignores what is presented in this book and still does not allow the *protective wall* of evidence-based medicine, with its claims according to controlled randomized trials, to be broken through.

There are also different safe research methods, other than just the commonly propagated large clinical trials. Empirical medicine, with well-documented case descriptions, naturalistic studies, and findings from studies on animals and cell cultures, can certainly make a scientific statement about the effect of a treatment method.

But this way of researching is still not well-known and not promoted and has so far been ignored by the *global players*. The content presented here makes it easy to understand why this is the case.

For anyone who wants to get a better understanding of knowledge-based medicine as a new scientific route and thus delve deeper into the treatment methods presented in this book, the *Zeitschrift für ärztliche Fortbildung* (German Journal for Continuous Medical Education) from 2005 with the title "What Is Cognition-Based Medicine?" is recommended, as well as the following website: www.ifaemm.de.

The Institute for Applied Epistemology and Medical Methodology at the Witten-Herdecke University in Germany also provides information.

Chapter Two

How the Light Shines

In the beginning there was light! All life as we know it, understand it, and can imagine it came into being through the influence of the sun on our planet.

When it comes to the significance of the sun for life on earth, we find the often-quoted passage in Herbert Friedman's book *The Sun* (1997) apt: "The sun sustains all life on earth, it illuminates us, warms the ground, the oceans, the atmosphere, it controls the climate, it brings droughts and ice ages, it drives the wind that blows across the earth and determines our weather. Its storms interfere with radio communication, cause electrical damage and even mark the rings of trees with radioactivity."

The sun is constantly converting hydrogen into helium in its interior as part of a process that has lasted billions of years. In doing so, an incredible amount of energy is released, which in turn triggers countless chemical and physical processes. Plant life, animal life, and human life would not exist without the sun, nor would any other form of life. But the significance of the sun for our lives and our globe goes even further. All complex atoms, from which we and nature surrounding us are formed, originated from the processes of atomic fusion of hydrogen in the core of the sun, as modern astrophysics has established. From the point of view of modern astrophysics, the sun is a gigantic, energy-releasing nuclear reactor in the center of our solar system.

The exploration and scientific study of light in cells of all organisms began about 150 years ago with the Russian biologist and physician Alexander Gurwitsch (1874–1954). As a histologist, he was concerned with the science of biological tissues and made an astonishing discovery in 1923: While studying the cell division of onion cells, he was able to detect a faint glow in the ultraviolet wavelength at 260 nanometers, a range of light radiation that the naked human eye can no longer perceive. He suspected that this light originated from the biochemical processes of cell division, and therefore called it mitogenetic radiation (*mitosis* means "cell division").

Today, his discovery is known as ultraweak photon emission, and it occurs as a result of chemical reactions. It can be measured only with a special apparatus, a photomultiplier, and is only just above the technical detection limit. The photon emission must not be confused with bioluminescence—for example, as in the case of fireflies.

In ancient Greek, *photon* means "light." In physics, photons are light quantities and physically the smallest units of light. They are called biophotons when they are emitted by living cells.

Although Gurwitsch correctly assumed—as many scientists still do today—that this radiation could stimulate mitosis (division of the cell nucleus) of cells, after initial recognition, his research was soon questioned and dismissed as unimportant.

Today, it is assumed that the glow is not only a result of chemical reactions, but could also be a response to external influences or internal damage, which could be caused by toxic substances, such as chemicals or substances excreted by microorganisms. However, photon emission can possibly also change due to physical influences such as extreme temperatures, radiation, and electricity, and also due to mechanical effects.

The German biophysicist and professor Fritz-Albert Popp (1938–2018) confirmed Gurwitsch's observations by measurements with light amplifiers and thereby became one of the founders of the aforementioned biophotonics, which today is a distinct branch of science dealing with the phenomenon of cellular luminosity and its possible significance.

Although the existence of biophotons is now undisputed, some of Popp's research, probably like Gurwitsch's at the time, was also rejected by established science. These reactions also indicate a certain explosiveness. After all, Popp was researching no lesser question than what life is.

To this day, the topic of biophotons and their significance is controversially discussed. Despite numerous publications, it has not found universal recognition in the established world of mainstream science. As a form of neovitalism, it is derided or rejected by its critics as a field of interest of the alternative-esoteric scene, while other scientists and colleagues regard Popp as a very competent scientist who has broken new ground with his research and findings.

Outside the realm of popular science, biophotonics has been met with great interest among scientists and physicians who are concerned with alternative concepts and consider intercellular communication with the help of light based on chemical processes to be possible.

With Popp's experimental setup, sick cells can be differentiated from healthy cells by the pattern of light they emit, and his statement, "Cancer is a kind of communication disturbance in the subtle signals which the cells use to communicate with one another," could be a further step toward answering the questions of how and why cancer develops and how cancer can be treated.

Popp's experiments with living and dead cells showed that in living systems (without renewed energization by sunlight), the photon radiation subsides more slowly than in inanimate systems. Living cells glow more intensely and for longer than dead cells, which do continue to emit a fundamentally weaker light for some time, but whose light then also "goes out" more quickly.

Biophotons are produced by electrons, which are in turn stimulated by sunlight, Popp concluded. For him, this was the proof that the electrons of a living organism or a recently picked plant inform one another, that is, they are in exchange with one another at the speed of light. The light that these cells emit is, like a laser, also coherent. Coherent light is highly ordered and has the same wavelength, or color, and the same orientation of the waves with their crests and troughs. It therefore appears collimated and clearly aligned.

For us, however, this phenomenon is also a bridge between philosophy and science, between vital field hypothesis and measurable biophysics. It has its relevance, for example, in the quality research of foodstuffs and also in the treatment of diseases with coherent light, the above-mentioned laser light.

The quality of food, for example, can be determined by measuring light emissions. The more light a product can store and then release, the fresher and healthier it is, as a rule. Light measurement provides evidence that is not accessible with conventional methods. In experiments, eggs from conventional farming stored significantly less light than those from organic farming. The same phenomenon can be seen when examining organically produced fruit, vegetables, or meat. According to Popp, the difference lies in the "order of the substances," and the light storage capacity can be seen as a measure of the degree of organization of the cell. True to the motto "You are what you eat," it seems to be sensible and healthy—with a coherence-based way of life—to eat those foods that are characterized by a higher degree of vitality, or a greater order of substances.

Apart from the *added value* that our body can obviously benefit from in this way, we also increase the coherence of other systems and areas of life by promoting and consuming organically produced products. The biophoton emission shows a connection between the vitality and well-being of an organism.

These coherently glowing cells represent an order, which—if we consume them—can in turn help to create more order in our organism. The higher degree of organization equals higher quality and higher vitality.

According to Popp, healthy cells emit coherent light, while cancer cells emit noncoherent, chaotic-seeming light. In relation to cancer—or other diseases—the promotion of coherence is therefore a universally therapeutic principle of stimulating the chaotically growing cells to redifferentiate, to redevelop into normal cells by increasing the coherent order in an organism.

This is the aim of nontoxic cancer treatments and the principle of action through treatment with a variety of biological anticancer agents (see chapter 6) in order to restimulate the lost apoptosis—the natural death of cancer cells—that characterizes all healthy cells. A healthy cell has a certain lifespan and dies a natural cell death when it becomes too old, which is called apoptosis.

A cancer cell is no longer able to do this. It is potentially "immortal" and will perish only when the entire organism around it decays and dies.

The less coherent the complex life processes of a cell are, the less differentiated the cell is and the more aggressive its cancerous nature. However, the more a cancer cell returns to the coherent rhythm of life, the more highly differentiated it is and the slower it grows into cancerous tumors in an organism.

Since a complete elimination of cancer cells in virtually all cases of metastatic cancers appears not to be possible, the aim should be to turn them into inactive cancer cells, so-called dormant cancer, as Japanese scientists found in 2019. The aim is therefore to influence or even cure the cancer cells that survive as a remainder after a successful therapy, by increasing coherence in such a way that they turn into dormant cancer cells with which the organism can live in balance and grow old.

In his book *Biophotons: The Light in Our Cells*, Marco Bischof describes that cancer represents the entire organism's loss of coherence and light storage capacity. While it seems healthy cells can store light better, the opposite is true with malignant cancer cells: the more uncontrolled and rapid their multiplication is, the more light they radiate. Popp was able to confirm with human tumor cells what had already been discovered experimentally by Dennis Schamhart from the University of Utrecht in 1983–1984. Schamhart and his colleagues were able to measure that cancer cells have a less coherent light pattern than healthy cells, that they behave in a more disordered manner. This means that the ability to form a meaningful collective with other cells, called *syncytium*, is lost.

A tumor tissue consists of autistically behaving cells that cannot contribute to a higher whole, but rather all live individually at the development level of a single-cell organism. Here, it becomes visible again (similar to what is shown in section 3.9, "Mitochondria: Power Plants of the Cells," on page 125) that the cancer cell has taken a big step backward in the evolution of life. The ability to form syncytia is an achievement of higher life forms, where many cells come together to form a *higher whole* and where each cell takes into account the "common good" of the whole organism and thus subordinates itself to it.

We regard this as an expression of an ordering field of life, since no scientific explanation can be found in the whole of biology as to what actually causes this ability to live together in a more highly organized cell association.

Likewise, the phenomenon of the organ and organism form is difficult to understand or cannot be understood at all with the concepts of the current doctrine of biology alone. Here, too, we see a need to leave behind the narrow framework of the reductionist cell biology based on biochemistry and to think in the dimension of *vital fields*, as the English biochemist Rupert Sheldrake described in his work: It is "morphogenetic fields" that are at work here.

Popp postulated a chaos-coherence control circuit controlled by biophotons, which is derailed in its growth regulation when cancer occurs. Accordingly, the cancer problem is not the tumor, but the lost regulatory capacity of the organism as a whole. According to Popp, tumors are late and only locally occurring symptoms.

The findings of Gurwitsch, Popp, Budwig (see also section 3.2, "Healthy Nutrition and Health-Promoting Dietary Supplements Using the Example of the Twelve Vital Fields," on page 36), and other scientists also concur in the research on mitochondria. The mitochondria, known as *power plants of the cell*—more details in section 3.9, "Mitochondria: Power Plants of the Cell," on page 125—are highly responsible for our health and our quality of life.

Despite sufficient research, however, this topic still receives far too little attention in conventional medicine.

Biophoton analysis is not only a measuring instrument for the vital force of living cells, but it can also illuminate a connection between the ancient ideas of life force/prana/chi and physically measurable energy. For example, in the paraphrasing of aura, prana (India), or chi (China), we see philosophical-vitalist concepts, the understanding of which is, at its core, revitalization and maintenance as well as the recognition of a divine spark in everything.

Popp's statement that light is a signal carrier brings us full circle with the realization that everything is connected by a huge network of light and energy and that the light in our cells is not only to enable communication between the cells, but also to communicate with all other systems and even with a divine life force. This is the holistic principle.

The *Great Hymn to the Aton* by the Egyptian Pharaoh Akhenaten, for example, already refers to the life-giving force of the sun and the unique significance of its light for life on earth. There it states, among other things:

> *Thou appearest beautifully on the horizon of heaven,*
> *Thou living Aton, the beginning of life!*
> ...
> *How manifold it is, what thou hast made!*
> *They are hidden from the face (of man).*
> *O sole god, like whom there is no other!*
> *Thou didst create the world according to thy desire,*
> *Whilst thou wert alone: All men, cattle, and wild beasts,*
> *Whatever is on earth, going upon (its) feet,*
> *And what is on high, flying with its wings.*
>
> —AKHENATEN, circa 1351–1334 BC

In a poem by Goethe ("Zahme Xenien"), it is also made clear in a poetic way how the sun and man, God and that which delights us, is based on the principle of resonance. Like attracts like, like causes like to resonate, or figuratively, to delight. Life shines because it is born of light. And like an echo, a reverberation of the beginning of all life from the energy of the sunlight, it shines in all our cells, as long as they live and we live with them.

> *The eye must be something like the sun,*
> *Otherwise no sunlight could be seen;*
> *God's own power must be inside us,*
> *How else could Godly things delight us?*[2]
> —JOHANN WOLFGANG VON GOETHE (1749–1832)

Chapter Three

The Holistic Model of the Twelve Vital Fields

3.1 The Detoxification of the Organism

All things are poison and nothing is without poison—
the dosage alone makes it
so a thing is not a poison.

—Paracelsus

This rather common phrase was penned by the doctor and natural scientist Philippus Theophrastus Bombast von Hohenheim, better known as Paracelsus, who lived from 1493 to 1541. The concept and result of his extensive research was *sola dosis fazit venenum* (only the dose makes the poison).

Paracelsus was born in 1493 in Einsiedeln in what is now Switzerland. After completing his doctorate in Ferrara, he traveled through various countries for several years before becoming a town doctor in Basel. Today, he is considered one of the forefathers of modern pharmacy. Paracelsus recognized early on that toxins in our body are those substances that are present in too high a concentration or quantity.

Today more than ever, these can be substances of various origins that we ingest or have ingested in too high a quantity and that we are unable to egest, or detoxify, in corresponding quantities.

The topic of toxin load or detoxification of the body also leads us back to the state of health as a balance between toxification and detoxification. Every day we consume substances that are potentially toxic, such as pesticides, preservatives in food, heavy metals such as lead and mercury, chemical substances from body care products, cosmetics, and clothing, and in addition, the air pollution in many cities takes its toll on our organism. However, as long as we can get rid of these substances again and the body's detoxification mechanisms function well and are not overburdened, toxins do not necessarily have to make us ill. Being healthy therefore requires us, on the one hand, not to exceed a tolerable level of toxin intake and, on the other hand, to keep the body's own detoxification methods going or, if necessary, to activate them. Toxins that challenge or even overtax our organism can be divided into three categories.

3.1.1 Environmental Toxins

The first category includes environmental toxins, which we absorb by breathing, eating, and drinking, or through our skin, but which our organism does not need for its biochemical processes, the constructive and breakdown processes.

Small quantities of these environmental toxins can be compensated for daily by a healthy organism—they can be detoxified and excreted. Larger quantities, however, overtax the organism and its detoxification capacity. The toxins that are not broken down and excreted accumulate over time and increasingly block the important biochemical processes in the body, which in turn leads to the formation of further secondary toxins.

A good example of this is pathological liver detoxification. If the detoxification capacity of the liver is exceeded, toxic substances are produced in it that additionally burden and damage the organism. This creates a cycle with negative feedback, which is very significant for the vitality of the organism. It can no longer help itself and should be treated and supported with, for example, milk thistle, sulfur-containing amino acids, bile-boosting agents, and orthomolecular medicine.

Examples of common environmental toxins are heavy metals, spraying agents, artificial fertilizers, agricultural pesticides, exhaust fumes, fine dust, household cleaning agents, vapors from technical equipment (for example, flame retardants), and chemical residues from textiles, paints, and the like.

3.1.2 **Organically Developed Toxins**

The second group of toxins includes substances that are—when ingested in the right quantity—either harmless or even perform an important task in our body. Technically, they are not (yet) toxins. Only when they are ingested in excessive quantities do they become toxic and damage the organism.

We find toxins of this kind in our unhealthy diet today in the form of too much sugar and too much animal fat, but also too many dairy products and carbohydrates and too much alcohol or gluten overload the organism. It is important to find the right amount for each person and, in the case of illness, to relieve the burden by abstaining from certain nutrients.

The toxins in our body are the result of a metabolism that is out of balance. An excess of sugar and meat consumption makes the body *acidic*. These acids become toxins when they exceed a healthy level and are no longer in balance with the corresponding alkaline substances.

A good example of this is the breakdown of alcohol in the liver. The liver is responsible for about 95–98 percent of the alcohol breakdown, while only a very small portion of the alcohol is broken down by means of the lungs, skin, and kidneys.

The breakdown process of alcohol in the liver causes—among other things—toxic acetaldehyde to be produced from the ethanol. The acetaldehyde is converted into acetate (acetic acid), released into the body fluids via the liver, and is eventually transformed into carbon dioxide and water. Finally, the toxins are excreted through breath, sweat, and urine.

One can therefore imagine that not just alcohol consumption in moderation, but especially regular and excessive alcohol consumption leads or can lead to the liver being greatly burdened and poisoned. The situation is similar with uric acid, which is produced, among other things, by the breakdown of animal proteins in the liver and small intestine. If there is also a small excretion via the kidneys, it is deposited in the joints and, in extreme cases, leads to painful gout.

3.1.3 **Medicines as Toxins**

A third, very special category of toxins are medicines. Alarmingly, they are one of the common causes of death today. The main cause of kidney failure, for example, is the excessive use of painkillers, which in many cases requires lifelong dialysis treatment—*dialysis* refers to blood-washing treatment with an artificial kidney—or a kidney transplant. In hospitals, death due to drug side effects has been ranked the fourth most common cause of death for many years. It is estimated that in Germany alone, between thirty thousand and sixty thousand people die every year as a result of taking too high a dose or too much of a drug, albeit taken exactly as prescribed by their doctor. According to US statistics from 2009, more people died because of medicines than were killed in road accidents.

This phenomenon was investigated by Andreas Sönnichsen, head of the Institute of General Medicine and Family Medicine at the University of Witten-Herdecke, in a small pilot study with 169 patients from twenty-two general practices, which was reported on in 2013. As well as dosing errors and interactions between medications, it was found that for two-thirds of polypharmacy patients (patients who are treated with many medications at the same time), there was no scientific justification for prescribing certain medications.

Similarly, a 2017 European Union study of around four thousand patients and over three hundred general practitioners (GPs) found that almost one in three medicines was unsuitable for the respective patient for a variety of reasons. These reasons included relevant interactions with other medications and incorrect dosages. According to Sönnichsen, it is not only unsuitable medicines that are prescribed, but also often those whose side effects are not recognized or are misinterpreted. As a result, side effects are often interpreted as a new, independent illness and are in turn treated with another drug.

In Germany, the statutory health insurance providers are obliged to offer "general practitioner–centered care" (HzV, *"Hausarztzentrierte Versorgung"*) to their policyholders. However, this GP model is voluntary for the GPs and their patients (in general: the policyholders). Except for emergencies and visits to gynecologists, ophthalmologists, dentists, and pediatricians, patients should always contact their GP first for questions regarding health problems, so that they can take over the treatment (which should save additional costs) and, if necessary, refer them to specialists and hospitals. Above all, an overview of the patient's medical history and the treatment carried out, including the medication taken, can be maintained. Ideally, this avoids medication errors and overmedication with undesired interactions and damage to health. If a

GP offers this model and the patients want to make use of it, they must agree to see their GP first for a year.

For recovery as well as for staying healthy, it is of great importance to keep the toxin load in the organism and its detoxification capacity in balance or to bring it back into balance by intensifying and optimizing the detoxification activity.

The four important detoxification organs that need to be strengthened, not least in chronic illnesses and cancer, are the liver with its production of bile, the kidneys with their urine production, the mucous membranes and the peristalsis (ability to move) of the digestive tract, and the sweat glands of the skin.

In addition to a healthy lifestyle—which ideally consists of a wholesome, organic diet, regular exercise in the countryside or sports activity out in the fresh air, social contacts, such as family and friendships, and meaningful occupational activity, and which should not be associated with too much negative stress—there are various therapeutic measures to improve the detoxification capacity of the body. These include liver-activating substances such as milk thistle, B vitamins, and antioxidants (selenium, vitamin C, zinc, and others), as well as sulfur-containing substances such as L-cysteine, MSM (methylsulfonylmethane, a sulfur-containing food supplement), and glutathione (a tripeptide, which is the body's own sulfur-containing molecule consisting of three amino acids and is found in almost all cells).

In order to provide the body with sulfur-containing compounds and anti-inflammatory substances against chronic inflammation and cancer through food, all types of cruciferous vegetables can be consumed.

Although the different types of cruciferous vegetables look very different, they are very similar in their composition of carbohydrates, fats, and proteins, and high content of various vitamins, minerals, and fibers.

They all belong to the cabbage family, which, among other things, produces detoxifying sulfur compounds. These substances are counted among the secondary plant substances and are summarized as glucosinolates. There are about 120 of these sulfur-containing compounds that have been shown to inhibit cancer growth and enhance the effect of chemotherapy.

The vitalizing and detoxifying foods and their effects are described in more detail in section 3.2, "Healthy Nutrition and Health-Promoting Dietary Supplements Using the Example of the Twelve Vital Fields," on page 36).

The Detoxifying Effect of Fever

The ability to induce fever is one of the most ingenious inventions of the evolution of higher mammals and humans. It serves not only to fire up the immune system in the fight against invading microorganisms, but also to improve the detoxification of the organism via the sweat glands. The beneficial and health-promoting effect of the sauna is partly based on this mechanism. Sweating during sports also has a detoxifying effect, and anyone who wants to ward off a cold coming on would do well to take an overheated bath. This can raise the body temperature by a good 1°C. Afterward, it is best to drink two cups of hot elderberry tea, which encourages sweating even more, then to lie down in bed and sleep: Our immune systems are particularly active when we are asleep. Quite often, you can already notice that the cold is significantly better by the morning after these activities.

Brush Massage

The pores of our skin, both the sweat glands and the sebaceous glands, can be cared for and kept open by gently massaging and brushing them, using a proper massage brush, from the periphery of the arms and legs inward toward the heart. Three minutes of dry brushing in the morning not only gets the lymphatic flow going, but also encourages the natural detoxification of the skin.

Coffee Enemas According to Dr. Gerson

Another method for increasing detoxification, particularly by stimulating the bile activity, is the coffee enema according to the German-American doctor Max Gerson (1881–1959). Gerson used the caffeine and numerous antioxidants contained in coffee to improve the liver's detoxification capacity.

Today we know that coffee has a whole range of health-promoting properties. The antioxidant effect of various constituents reduces the risk of elevated liver values, liver cirrhosis, and liver cell cancer. In general, coffee improves detoxification by stimulating the formation of detoxification enzymes.

But with coffee, too, the dosage is crucial. Drunk in moderation—we recommend two to three cups a day, preferably espresso roast and preparation with little acidity—coffee is a potential anticancer agent.

But why also as an enema? The explanation is related to the blood supply of the rectum with its direct connection to the liver. If we take coffee as an enema in the form of approximately seven hundred to eight hundred milliliters of liquid through the rectum, it is fed directly into the liver via enterohepatic circulation, which is the direct blood connection between the rectum and the liver. The quantity of coffee substances absorbed in the liver in this way is much higher than what we absorb in the liver by conventional drinking, because when we drink it, the coffee substances are carried throughout the entire body before they reach the liver.

Since 2014, the effect of coffee has been intensively researched, and the US National Cancer Institute was able to show in a published study that coffee consumption improves the merits of various liver enzymes.

This means that patients with chronic liver inflammation can also benefit from coffee. In 2015, Japanese researchers from the Japanese National Institute of Infectious Diseases demonstrated in laboratory experiments that, for example, caffeic acid can inhibit the multiplication of hepatitis C viruses.

––––––––––

Our conclusion: Moderate espresso consumption is healthy, and for illnesses associated with toxicity, a coffee enema is beneficial. We recommend to our patients with liver strain (with elevated liver values, liver metastases, liver cancer, or after liver-straining chemotherapy) a series of coffee enemas: three times on consecutive days, preferably in the morning, and then once or twice a week as needed until the condition improves. We are not aware of any side effects.

3.2 Healthy Nutrition and Health-Promoting Dietary Supplements Using the Example of the Twelve Vital Fields

Is there an *anticancer diet*? And what does *healthy eating* mean?

While we are inundated with a flood of different diets for all sorts of purposes and circumstances, it is difficult to search for the dietary lifestyle that will eliminate all evils that make us ill, without seeking professional advice or help. The more extreme and one-sided such a diet is shown to be and the more it promises great miracles in a short period of time, the more skeptical we should be. Nutrition is a fundamental, very emotional subject that is influenced by many personal, cultural, religious, geographic, age-related, and habitual circumstances, and by physical and genetic conditions, among other things.

Nutrition depends on our origins and upbringing, on our financial situation, where we live and our living situation, our social environment, time, and more and more frequently on fashions and health trends, which are changing more and more quickly, inventing new things or rediscovering forgotten ones.

While we as dietary life (stage) forms cannot choose a *one size fits all* approach, but should decide and adjust individually, it is easier with healthy nutrition: We can discuss what is healthy and what the body needs to be healthy, meaning resilient and a good home for the psyche, in general terms. Indeed, an old saying goes: "Food keeps body and soul together," but what kind of food is meant, and what kind of eating behavior and which foodstuffs help to do this? The following is an overview, in terms of the twelve vital fields, of foods, micronutrients, vitamins, minerals, trace elements, fatty acids, and influential food supplements that deserve our special attention.

A healthy diet is characterized by variety and by finding out personal needs and preferably approaching the broad topic of nutrition with curiosity, openness, and, of course, some time. There are many examples of diets that claim to be able to "cure" cancer, but there is no clear evidence.

In the maze of different dietary recommendations, it is difficult to find the one or the only right way. Does it exist at all? The Gerson diet, the Breuss juice fast, the vegan diet, the paleo diet, the ketogenic diet, the alkaline diet, and intermittent fasting are just a few examples. Some of these diets, when used optimally and practiced for a limited period of time, can improve the vitality of the organism. However, if extreme diets are followed for too long, they can also be dangerous, especially for a weakened organism.

The purpose of nutrition is to provide our body with as much vitality and energy as necessary, so that the complex occurrence of *life* in our approximately sixty quadrillion cells with about fifteen quintillion biochemical reactions every second can take place in the best possible way.

The basic rule for a healthy diet is to include as many fruits and vegetables in our daily menu as possible. Of course, our food should be as natural as possible and not processed (preserved, sweetened with sugar, chemically treated, etc.). It is always advisable to use organically produced fruits and vegetables, because otherwise we try to eat healthily in one way and, for example, want to get rid of toxins, but we are ingesting them in another way.

In general, a healthy diet is low in toxins, is anti-inflammatory and detoxifying, contains about ninety essential nutrients (minerals, vitamins, amino acids, fatty acids, micronutrients, and trace elements), includes sufficient intake of fresh water, and promotes optimal oxygen utilization in the body.

For example, the main focus of the so-called Budwig diet is a special mixture of polyunsaturated fatty acids from linseed and proteins containing sulfhydryl (e.g., in quark or cottage cheese), which is supposed to reoxygenate, or supply with oxygen, and restore the function of damaged cells (this is a direct link to our discussion in chapter 2, and also section 3.9, "Mitochondria: Power Plants of the Cells," on page 125).

Healthy eating means eating in peace, without rushing and without stress. It is good for the intestinal flora, is low in rapidly utilizable carbohydrates (i.e., low-carb), promotes the physiological acid–base balance, and is free from pathogenic microorganisms.

This means that a healthy diet does not avoid carbohydrates altogether, as some diets would have us believe, but it certainly reduces carbohydrates and, if grains are used, they should be whole grains that are simultaneously also rich in dietary fibers. A healthy diet also contains very specific components that the mitochondria of our cells need (L-carnitine and selenium, among others) and holistically supports the immune system.

But in order to find out what a healthy diet consists of, let us look at the vital field with its twelve fields in detail. Although it is important to have a diverse and fresh—and seasonal—variety, a few particular "nutritional artists" are highlighted in the following.

Each individual theme of the twelve vital fields is equally related to those of the other fields of this system and—although numbered for our purposes and for better structuring—can be exchanged for any other and change its place in the overall structure.

The order of the individual vital fields is not to be imagined as if they build on one another or have a hierarchy. The entire vital field with its twelve individual fields arises from the systemic thinking that everything is connected to and permeated by everything else. If we change our behavior and habits in one field, this will also and automatically have an effect in one or more other fields.

3.2.1 The Anti-Inflammatory Diet

Inflammation, in addition to the positive effect of fighting infections and expelling unwanted substances from the body, has the disadvantage of being able to establish itself chronically in the organism. Even it if does not appear so at first glance, Crohn's disease, rheumatism, arthritis, gastritis (inflammation of the gastric mucosa), depression, cancer, and asthma have something in common: They can be brought about by inflammation, or they can worsen as a result of inflammation. The anti-inflammatory diet is a fresh and varied mixed diet with a significantly high proportion of plant-based foods, which include some particularly effective types of plants and fatty acids.

Cruciferous Vegetables

Besides leafy vegetables in general, with their numerous antioxidants and a large amount of vitamins and phytochemicals, a very important but completely underestimated vegetable is cabbage. The German were often, and not always without malice, nicknamed "The Krauts" abroad (sauerkraut was originally part of central European [food] culture and eaten in many variations and situations).

Thanks to various innovations and fashions since the 1950s, thanks to fast food and globalization, Germans have managed to largely distance themselves from this pet name. So it is all the more gratifying that, due to research and the latest health movements, the joy of cabbage has been rediscovered with recipes that have been dusted off—both raw and fermented as well as cooked.

All types of cabbage belong to the cruciferous family and have glucosinolates in common. Briefly mentioned in the previous chapter as part of the phytochemicals, glucosinolates are chemical compounds that contain sulfur and nitrogen and are formed from amino acids. In their chemical mode of action, they are an important aspect of oxygenation, or oxygen enrichment in the tissue, while in terms of taste, they give all representatives of the cruciferous family their typical pungent and bitter flavor. In the case of mustard, cress, nasturtium, radish, and horseradish, the pungent-bitter note is usually more pronounced than in many types of cabbage.

Since children still have a strongly developed sense of taste for bitter substances, it is not surprising that they sometimes react with great aversion to the sharpness of cress or the bitter aroma of Brussels sprouts.

To get the full benefit of the oxygenating substances, cabbage should be cut into pieces before being cooked and left to air for a while, since the plant cells consist of two chambers: one contains the glucosinolate, the other contains an enzyme called myrosinase. If the cabbage is damaged (by cutting, breaking, or biting), these two substances come into contact with each other and only then form the various mustard oils whose effect is so healthy. They are actually used by the plant as a defense against predators.

In addition to glucosinolates, cabbage vegetables also contain many other phytochemicals, including the flavonoids (water-soluble plant pigments) quercetin and kaempferol, which play a special role in the context of therapies against cancer. They have a strong anti-inflammatory and antioxidant effect on free O_2 radicals in the body—a chemically overactive and therefore potentially harmful variation of oxygen—and also anti-allergic, antiviral (virus-killing), antimicrobial (bacteria- and parasite-killing), and anticarcinogenic (cancer-inhibiting) properties.

Cabbage vegetables are also rich in vitamins. Particularly important here are the B-group vitamins, vitamins C and K, and beta-carotene. While broccoli and Brussels sprouts contain the most vitamin C, Brussels sprouts also top the table in terms of vitamin K content. Minerals such as calcium, magnesium, potassium, iron, and copper are also abundant.

As one of the vegetables richest in fiber, cabbage especially contributes to intestinal health and is the best preventive against disease and inflammation. How a diet rich in fiber contributes to detoxification is explained in section 3.2.2, "Detoxifying Substances in Food," on page 46, under dietary fibers.

Onion Family

The onion family includes, among others, onions, spring onions, leeks, shallots, chives, garlic, and wild garlic. Members of the onion family have always been valued for their antibacterial effect and have been used to prevent or treat infectious diseases. They also have a high content of flavonoids—including the anticancer substance quercetin—and many amino acids containing sulfur and nitrogen. The alliin contained in the tubers and cloves is converted into allicin by enzymes when they are cut, which releases the essential oils and causes the typical smell—but also the weeping.

Allicin and its other degradation products, including above all ajoene, inhibit the growth of bacteria and fungi and have an antiviral effect. The sulfurous amino acids also inhibit the agglutination of blood platelets and thus prevent the formation of blood clots. Ajoene also has a strong influence on platelet accumulation, similar to the effect of aspirin, and has a blood-thinning effect. Overall blood circulation is improved by the consumption of onions, garlic, chives, and the like, and cardiovascular diseases are thus prevented.

The abundant quercetin has an antioxidant effect and helps the body to defend itself against aggressive free oxygen radicals. It has an anticarcinogenic and antimicrobial effect and is heat-stable, such that even fried onions still contain a high portion of it.

In contrast to the various types of cabbage vegetables, the high fructose content in vegetables of the onion family is responsible for the fact that we taste a pronounced sweet note in addition to the pungency. Unlike cabbage, however, we should not store onions cut for later use, not even in the refrigerator. Due to their antibiotic effect, they attract and absorb toxins from the environment like a magnet. Thus, half an onion kept for the next meal would bring toxins into our food that we actually wanted to get rid of by means of the healthy tuber's properties.

In terms of flavor, vegetables in the onion family definitely bring spice and depth to our dishes. If you want to avoid the smell, especially of garlic, you'll just have to grin and bear it, since despite all the home remedies and traditions, milk, parsley, and coffee beans don't really help against the strong smell. It literally permeates through all pores. But we can console ourselves: This is exactly what makes garlic and onions so healthy and effective!

Sufficient Omega-3 Fatty Acids

To relieve the organism and prevent inflammation, you should eat only small amounts of red meat (beef, veal, mutton, lamb, and rabbit) and no pork at all. Pork is notable for its high content of the fatty acid arachidonic acid, which promotes inflammatory processes in the organism.

Arachidonic acid is an unsaturated fatty acid from the group of omega-6 fatty acids and is found in many animal products, for example, meat, offal, eggs, lard, butter, and other dairy products. It is important for the immune system, but, as already mentioned, too much of the substance has the opposite effect. Inflammatory skin diseases, rheumatism, and gout are the result if we consume too many omega-6 fatty acids and too few omega-3 fatty acids.

Marine and vegetable omega-3 fatty acids, on the other hand, have a demonstrably positive effect on the vitality of our cells. However, apart from the moral and ethical question, which each person must figure out for themselves, the consumption of fish—just like that of meat—is, due to intensive animal farming and the associated administration of medicines, overfishing the oceans, and environmental pollution, for example, by heavy metals, not *just* to be regarded as healthy. Ten milliliters of fish oil per day (also available in capsule form) should be consumed. But for the reasons just mentioned, these food supplements should come only from protected sources.

Fats and their importance are discussed in more detail in section 3.2.5, "Oxygen Saturation in the Cells," on page 52. This connection is also dealt with in more detail in section 3.4, "Oxygen, Breathing, and Cancer Growth," on page 82, and section 3.9, "Mitochondria: Power Plants of the Cells," on page 125.

Fruits

As mentioned above, the fruits in our diet should be as varied as possible. In different compositions, they are all rich in minerals, vitamins, trace elements, and fiber.

Pectin, which is predominantly contained in the peel in some fruits, can, for example, inhibit the proliferation of prostate, breast, and skin cancer. Where possible, fruits should be eaten with the skin on, since it is also rich in fiber and is good for digestion. In addition, the sugars in fruits do not enter the bloodstream as quickly if the fiber-rich peels also have to be digested. This benefits people with diabetes or with an intolerance: People who have a fructose or glucose intolerance, allergies, or diabetes, for example, should inform themselves as to which types of fruit are unsuitable and which are suitable for them as individuals.

If we look at the sugar (content) alone, what applies for fruits also applies to the various types of vegetables, since they, too, always contain glucose and fructose (see also section 3.2.2, "Detoxifying Substances in Food," on page 46, and dietary fibers in section 3.7, "Sugar: Cancer Driver of the First Order," on page 108).

It should be mentioned that intolerances and diabetes can be permanently positively influenced or even completely controlled by changing your diet. Depending on the severity, further medication can even become superfluous.

Particularly noteworthy among the various types of fruits are, for example, seasonal and locally grown berries, which have, among other things, anti-inflammatory, antibiotic, antioxidant, and detoxifying effects. If fresh berries are not available, some varieties can easily be dried and almost all berries can be frozen while keeping all the same health benefits when consumed.

Contrary to some beliefs, freezing does not have a damaging effect on vitamins, minerals, and health-promoting micronutrients. If fruits or vegetables are flash-frozen immediately after harvesting, the valuable goodness is retained with virtually no loss, and the cold even protects them from decay, which would otherwise occur during transport and storage. By withdrawing or freezing the water, the vitamin C and polyphenols, for example, are completely preserved and antioxidant substances remain up to 92 percent effective. Of course, the same does not apply to processed foods and ready-made frozen meals.

Stone fruits native to Germany and central Europe, as well as apples and pears, which belong to the rose family, are rich in health-promoting and disease-inhibiting substances. The old proverb "an apple a day keeps the doctor away" is so well-known that it is quoted all over the world in English or has found its way into the respective language. In Italy, for example, "una mela al giorno, toglie il medico di torno." Even in Chinese, the wisdom is expressed in a rhyme: "Yītiān yīgè píngguǒ, yīshēng yuǎnlí wǒ."

Scientific studies suggest that a diet rich in vitamin C plays a decisive role in cancer prevention. Among the tropical and citrus fruits, the lemon in particular should be a regular part of the diet. In addition to its vitamin C content, it is a fruit with many anticarcinogenic components that is particularly noteworthy—but only if it is eaten with the peel!

The peel contains the group of active substances called limonoids, which give all citrus fruits—but particularly lemons, where they are abundant—their bitter taste. These bitter substances have the property of slowing down cancer cell growth, lowering fever, and exerting antibacterial and antiviral properties, and in certain circumstances may even be able to eliminate cancer cells. Lemons are said to contain twenty-two anticancer compounds that can stop the cancer cells from dividing and reduce the risk of cancer by half, according to a 2016 *Natural News* report by the Commonwealth Scientific and Industrial Research Organisation of Australia.

The flavonoids contained in lemons not only have an anticancer effect, but also prevent heart attacks and improve the condition of our veins and arteries. The consumption of lemons also lowers blood lipid levels. The fact that abundant vitamin C strengthens the immune system in general and can prevent infectious illnesses is already known. However, vitamin C also plays an important role as a food supplement in high dosage in cancer therapy for cell renewal.

It is advisable to consume a whole lemon with the peel every day. Therefore, buy only organically grown fruit.

For some types of fruits and uses, it is recommended to freeze them after harvesting or purchasing them, in order to preserve their valuable goodness. Lemons can also be frozen—even just overnight—so that they can be grated whole the next day, including the peel, with a household grater. A lemon grated in this way can be used to infuse fresh water or added to a smoothie and is an ideal start to the day. However, the consumption of grapefruits, in particular, should be avoided during chemotherapy or radiotherapy, because they can considerably lower the effectiveness of these therapies.

The *lemon of the north*, sea buckthorn, is generally not as well known and tastes rather peculiar, but its vitamin C content is ten times higher than lemons.

Originally from the Himalayas, the family tree of the sea buckthorn goes back to the Ice Age. For almost all illnesses and health complaints, sea buckthorn can be used internally and externally. It is usually easily available in capsule form. In addition to vitamins B_1, B_6, E, and K, calcium, magnesium, and zinc, the small "nutrient bombs" also contain iron. If a content of vitamin B_{12} is indicated, which is found almost exclusively in animal products, this is in no case sufficient to meet the body's need for vitamin B_{12}. Sea buckthorn is rich in antioxidants and—used externally as well as internally—a true (almost) *all-rounder*.

More recently, pineapple and papaya have also been praised for containing the enzymes bromelain and papain. These enzymes have an anticarcinogenic effect and help to break down inflammatory proteins in the blood. However, it is difficult to obtain these acid-sensitive enzymes in sufficient concentrations through food alone—that is, through the stomach—especially since they are contained mainly in the unripe fruit or in the stalk and can withstand only stomach acid to a limited extent. Bromelain and papain are therefore also offered in special capsule or tablet form.

Anti-Inflammatory Food Supplements

TRYPSIN AND CHYMOTRYPSIN

Other anti-inflammatory dietary supplements in capsule or tablet form are protein-digesting enzymes (proteases), such as trypsin and chymotrypsin from animal pancreases.

The strongly colored yellow-orange spice turmeric is used in particular in Indian cuisine and in curries. The substance curcumin contained therein also has an anti-inflammatory effect. However, larger amounts of at least 1,125 to 2,500 milligrams of curcumin would need to be taken every day in order to achieve a noticeable anti-inflammatory effect, at least in the gastrointestinal tract. Due to the low absorption capacity for the fat-soluble curcumin from the intestine into the blood (less than 0.0001 percent), therapeutic or anti-inflammatory effects on the entire organism can be expected only very sparsely with orally ingested curcumin. For the treatment of illnesses such as cancer or inflammatory diseases, administration by intravenous infusion of curcumin is therefore much more effective (see also chapter 6).

For the prevention of inflammation in the intestine or for the treatment of milder forms of intestinal inflammation, high-dose preparations of curcumin are also available in capsule form, which are provided with a special emulsifier and thus achieve a bioavailability that is up to one hundred times higher.

FRANKINCENSE

The same applies to frankincense, which has strong anti-inflammatory properties and can even actively kill tumor cells. This happens through the boswellic acids contained in frankincense oil, which inhibit malignant tumor cells but do not affect healthy cells. In addition, frankincense taken orally in capsule form can alleviate the side effects of conventional cancer therapy and also has diuretic, digestive, and antiseptic effects. Here, too, it is important to take the right dose of boswellic acids in order to achieve the desired effect. Typical doses for oral frankincense therapy are 4.5–6 grams of *Boswellia serrata* powder per day, divided into three doses, or 1.5–2 grams three times a day. Recently, an injectable boswellia preparation called Bosvene has become available for clinical application, which has a significantly greater effect in the blood and thus in the whole organism.

GINGER

In addition to an anti-inflammatory effect, ginger also has active substances that attack and inhibit the proteins that normally protect cancer cells. In attacking the proteins, apoptosis (the "programmed" or natural cell death) of the cancer cell is induced; in other words, it dies a natural old age death just like a healthy cell.

While the body can develop resistance to drugs during breast cancer therapy, for example, this does not happen when taking ginger, which has no side effects. Ginger could ensure that cancer cells do not develop in the first place. It should therefore be taken habitually. As well as the natural consumption of ginger as a spice in food, there are also concentrated forms of ginger in capsules for oral intake.

In our practice, we have been routinely using an injectable form of ginger with the component 6-shogaol in the treatment of cancer patients for several years. Especially in breast cancer, 6-shogaol has made a name for itself as an effective herbal cytostatic in clinical studies.

3.2.2 Detoxifying Substances in Food

Dietary Fibers

As mentioned above, intestinal health is promoted by a diet rich in fiber. Apart from the fact that intestinal bacteria feed on fiber, they increase the intestinal contents, and they speed up intestinal movement. It could also be said that increased volume due to fiber stimulates the intestines to move the mass to be digested more actively. In this way, fewer harmful substances can be absorbed through the intestinal wall during this busy and vigorous process, and this in turn has a detoxifying effect on the organism.

Foods rich in fiber include all whole-grain products (they are always preferable to foods made from ground white flour!), vegetables and fruits, preferably with their skins, dried fruits, nuts, pulses, and other seeds. Dietary fibers can also be taken as a food supplement, for example, in the form of psyllium or acacia fiber, to promote detoxification of the organism.

We recommend a three-week course of treatment with an intestinal cleansing powder consisting of probiotics (healthy intestinal bacteria), fiber, and anti-inflammatory micronutrients at least once a year for healthy adults—and more frequently depending on the state of health. This powder is best taken in the evening, two hours after the last meal, stirred into about 200 milliliters of water. Afterward, taking another 150 milliliters of pure water should follow.

A diet rich in fiber promotes the health of the microbiome, or the natural composition of the many different intestinal bacteria (see also section 3.2.6, "The Healthy Microbiome," on page 57).

Lactic Acid Bacteria and Probiotics

Lacto-fermented vegetables, particularly sauerkraut, provide optimal support for intestinal health. The word *fermentation* is derived from the Latin word *fermentum*. The lactic acid bacteria and the enzymes already present on and in white cabbage are responsible for fermenting white cabbage into sauerkraut in the absence of oxygen at room temperature (around 20° C, or 68° F, or cooler). The microorganisms multiply on a huge scale and make sauerkraut— which is, just like all other lacto-fermented vegetables, a probiotic food.

It is precisely these lactic acid bacteria that are already part of our healthy intestinal environment and create a pleasant "comfortable climate" for useful intestinal bacteria, while pathogens have a very hard time in this environment. Probiotic foods therefore also help to build up a healthy intestinal flora. We should support our intestines especially during or after an illness, while or after taking medication—especially after antibiotics or chemotherapy with cytostatics—or while or after experiencing other stress, by consuming probiotic foods, so that toxins and pathogens are warded off as effectively as possible.

Other foods that are a result of fermentation include kimchi, tempeh, kombucha or kvass, and the well-known pickles. These are all helpful components of a healthy diet.

In the rediscovered and rather recent movement of pickling in lactic acid not only to preserve vegetables but also to make them particularly valuable for our health, there are hardly any limits; almost all types of vegetables are suitable.

If you do not want to ferment them yourself, you should make sure when buying sauerkraut and fermented vegetables (and vegetable juices) that they are fresh and not homogenized or pasteurized, because homogenization and pasteurization—neither of which is necessary for fermentation—both kill the valuable lactic acid bacteria in the food. Organic shops and supermarkets now offer lacto-fermented juices and lacto-fermented vegetables in bottles and jars year-round. Sauerkraut is also almost always available fresh, but especially during the winter cabbage season.

Sulfur

Sulfur is a chemical substance found, for example, in the amino acids cysteine, methionine, or the disulfide cystine, from which the body's own proteins are made. Sulfurous amino acids are important for healthy skin, tendons, bones, cartilage, and muscles and are an important component of connective tissue. Especially protein-containing foods, such as milk, eggs, yogurt, curd, cheese (especially Parmesan), fish, and meat, are rich in sulfur. However, we should be careful with the quantity and frequency of the foods we eat, since the (over)abundance of foods available to us nowadays means that we can have *too much of a good thing*, which can have the opposite effect.

The basic rule is to eat less meat and dairy, and eggs, poultry, and fish in moderation.

But nuts, garlic, rapeseed, wild garlic, mustard, onions, and pulses also contain many sulfurous amino acids. We do not generally consume these foods in overdosed quantities. On the contrary, the quantity of these foods can probably be increased for most of us for the benefit of our health.

With garlic, onions, wild garlic, radishes, and the like, we ingest sulfur compounds via alliin and the glucosinolates (see section 3.2.1, "Onion Family," on page 40), as well as through thiamine (vitamin B_1), biotin (vitamin B_7), and pantothenic acid (vitamin B_5).

The salts of the sulfuric acids, sulfates, play an important role in the detoxification of the organism, as together with water, harmful substances such as alcohol, arsenic, cadmium, and tobacco toxins are bound to them and excreted in urine.

Normally, our body is supplied with sufficient sulfur from our food.

However, for people with health problems, it can be advisable, particularly in the case of inflammatory diseases (such as arthrosis), to take additional sulfur supplements (for example, methylsulfonylmethane, MSM), as it not only relieves pain, but also has anti-inflammatory properties and helps to form new body cells.

Legumes

In Central European culture, legumes play a much smaller role than in their countries of origin in Asia, Africa, or South America, where they are very important as staple foods. In Europe, unfortunately, legumes often still have—like whole-grain products in general—a somewhat onerous eco-image.

The seeds of the legumes, which include peas, lentils, beans, soya beans, chickpeas, lupins, and peanuts, are not just beneficial for vegetarians and vegans. Of all plant foods, legumes have the highest protein content and are therefore essential for a strong immune system, which provides protection against germs and pathogens. The seeds of legumes are also characterized by a high-fiber content, the importance of which for intestinal health has already been briefly discussed.

Legumes are rich in natural, *good* carbohydrates. This is discussed in more detail in the sixth vital field under section 3.2.6, "The Healthy Microbiome," page 67.

We also find the vitamin thiamine (B_1) here. It has an important function for the nervous system and is colloquially known as the "mood vitamin." The metabolization of carbohydrates is one of its most important tasks, and it not only produces energy for the body but also detoxifies the body as effectively as possible.

Legumes also contain the minerals iron, potassium, and magnesium. Iron is not only necessary for the formation of red blood cells. It is also needed so that the blood cells can transport oxygen—bound to the iron-containing protein hemoglobin—in the blood, and thus ensure sufficient oxygen saturation of the cells.

Thus, in addition to breathing and exercise, we can also support our organism with the oxygenation of our tissues and cells by what we eat (see also section 3.4, "Oxygen, Breathing, and Cancer Growth," on page 82; section 3.9, "Mitochondria: Power Plants of the Cells," on page 125; and section 3.2.5, "Oxygen Saturation in the Cells," on page 52).

Special Micronutrients

Phytochemicals such as phytoestrogens, for example, from linseed, which are similar to the human sex hormone estrogen and have a positive effect in the prevention and complementary treatment of breast cancer, and phytosterols (mainly found in fat-rich plant parts; they are particularly abundant in sunflower seeds, wheat germ, sesame, soybeans, and pumpkin seeds) also have a positive effect on the body's cholesterol levels and thus prevent cardiovascular diseases and cancers.

Polyphenols

These occur as phytochemicals in many food plants and are bioactive substances (e.g., colorings, flavorings, and tannins) that protect the plant from predators. They are also anti-inflammatory and cancer-preventive, protect body cells from free radicals, and slow down cell oxidation. They are found in higher concentrations in the leaves and grapes of grapevines, but also in pomegranates, raspberries (in the form of ellagic acid), cistus, ginkgo, or green tea, all of which are rich in these health-promoting substances and contribute, among other things, to the optimal detoxification of our cells.

In natural doses, as they occur in the respective plants, polyphenols have positive biological properties. But in too high a dosage or through continuous use, they can have toxic effects: apigenin, quercetin, taxifolin, and kaempferol, for example, have a cytostatic effect (inhibiting cell division) and therefore should be used only in higher doses in a targeted manner and for a limited time. The polyphenol resveratrol has also gained special recognition. It is a highly effective antioxidant and can be found in vines, grapes, and red wine.

Detoxifying Food Substances

Milk thistle, selenium, and vitamin C are important detoxifying substances that can be taken as food supplements—individually or as combination preparations. They also contribute to the normal functioning of the immune system, protect the cells against oxidative stress, and help the liver to detoxify the whole organism. Milk thistle in particular, with the important compound silymarin, supports digestive function by stimulating the bile and the liver-bile system and also has an antioxidant and anti-inflammatory effect. For recommendations on the intake of food supplements for different personal circumstances with information on daily doses, see chapter 6.

3.2.3 The Balanced and Nutritious Diet

This part of the vital field includes all foods mentioned so far and the vitamins, minerals, antioxidants, fats, proteins, and much more contained therein.

In addition, fresh vegetables should of course be paramount in your diet, preferably untreated and organically grown: The shorter the delivery routes and storage times, the better and more *radiant* (see chapter 2) the vital properties of the food are for us. The more colorful the combination is, the better! This also results, quite incidentally, in an adaptation to seasonal availability. In this way, we not only support regional, natural cultivation, but we also do our organism good by making sure what we eat every day is as unprocessed as possible.

The seasonal menu often naturally offers exactly what our body particularly needs at that time. We noticeably feel that we have less of a craving for hearty foods like cabbage stew or sauerkraut in the summer than in the autumn and winter months. For example, the body demands a completely different availability of (warming) energy. The preparation—of the same food—can also be very different. Thus, in winter we might prefer to eat cooked beetroot, while in the summer we enjoy the same tubers as a raw vegetable salad. There are countless examples of this.

While there are winter and summer vegetables as well as winter and summer salads, they react differently to light conditions and temperatures—for example, root vegetables not only are easy to store and can be fermented without exception, they also are not influenced as much by personal and seasonal fluctuations.

In addition to daily fresh and colorful vegetables and root vegetables, fruits should of course also be featured in the diet. Nowadays, apart from the ecological (environmental) aspect, it is no longer a problem for us to choose from a vast selection of different types of fruit year-round.

This should include fresh berries. They have countless positive properties and can also be consumed frozen in winter, while other varieties (e.g., chokeberry) also make an important contribution to health when dried. Not only do they contain a wide variety of vitamins and minerals, and antioxidants, they also have antibiotic, detoxifying, anti-inflammatory, blood-forming and blood-cleansing, diuretic, digestive, immune-strengthening, draining, and metabolism-stimulating effects.

Colloquially, different species are grouped together as berries, and strawberries (although belonging to the aggregate nut fruit family) and blackberries and raspberries (belonging to the aggregate drupe fruit family) are mentioned in the same breath as, for example, currants, blueberries, lingonberries, gooseberries, bilberries, cranberries, rosehips, sea buckthorn, and elderberries.

Nuts and seeds should be consumed regularly. They are abundant in fibers, phytochemicals, and proteins. Lacto-fermented foods should also feature in our diet more often, as well as mushrooms from safe sources. Shiitake and maitake mushrooms are particularly recommended, also known and often used in Traditional Chinese Medicine. Among other things, mushrooms strengthen the intestinal immune system, promote the formation of T cells, and intensify the cytotoxic effect of the macrophages (the so-called *scavenger cells* or phagocytes) against pathogenic germs.

3.2.4 Drinking Enough Fresh Water

The fourth vital field reminds us to drink enough fresh water.

Water is the origin of all life—we have known that much for a long time. However, it is often underestimated how essential water is for the function of our cells—in particular, the case of mitochondria. That is why a whole section of this chapter is dedicated to the topic of water, its special characteristics and its effect on our organism and the preparation of tap water through swirling and filter systems (see section 3.3, "Water: An Elixir of Life," page 78). Here, suffice it to say: Remember to drink enough water, preferably, of course, fresh spring water.

3.2.5 Oxygen Saturation in the Cells

Fats and Their Importance for Our Nutrition

In order for life to evolve at all and health to be maintained in the best possible way, fats play an essential role.

Each of our cells is surrounded by fat molecules, the membrane lipids. Our brain and nerve cells contain fats, and all our organs are surrounded by a lipid layer (from the Greek *lipos*, meaning "fat"); the fat in fat molecules also act as important carriers of the fat-soluble vitamins A, D, E, and K.

Contrary to the widespread opinion that fat is unhealthy, and that the intake of fat (not least in order to stay slim or lose weight) should be avoided as far as possible, our body is actually dependent on the intake of fats through food. However, it matters how much and, above all, which fats we are talking about.

From a health point of view, we should avoid hydrogenated fats altogether. The so-called trans fats are artificially hardened fats that the body cannot process. They are found in processed foods (for example, margarine), ready-made meals, fast foods, industrially produced baked goods such as biscuits, pastries, and croissants, and potato chips and fried foods. They increase the risk of heart attack and even have negative effects on our brain.

Saturated Fatty Acids

In fact, we should be careful to eat saturated fats only in moderation. Not only because we can also produce them endogenously (within the body), but because too many can be harmful to our health.

They are mainly found in (processed) foods of animal origin, such as meat and sausage products, butter, cream, milk, palm oil, and cocoa butter.

Saturated fats primarily serve to provide the body with energy. But an excess of saturated fatty acids increases the levels of fat in the blood and thus increases the risk of cardiovascular diseases such as arteriosclerosis, thrombosis, angina pectoris, heart attacks, strokes, and aneurysms, as well as the risk of liver disease.

Cholesterol levels in the blood that are too high are generally (although often not specifically) treated with medication. More effective treatment, however, is a regulation of the levels through lifestyle changes that include the causes of the elevation. This has a positive effect on health in the long term.

Nowadays, most of our lifestyles are characterized by rushing and stress, little exercise, and no or hardly any physical work in the fresh air, as well as too few rest breaks and too little sleep. Too many animal products, highly processed foods, and ready-made meals are responsible for the fact that many of us consume more than the recommended daily amount of saturated fatty acids. In principle, fatty acids should not be more than one-third of the total amount of fats we consume per day, which, according to the German Nutrition Society, means no more than 7–10 percent of our daily energy intake.

However, there is one particularly health-promoting form of saturated fatty acid, namely coconut fat or coconut oil.

The difference in the names "fat" and "oil" is usually that many manufacturers distinguish between a natural virgin coconut "oil" with the (more or less pronounced) typical coconut taste and scent, and a deodorized coconut "fat." The typical taste and smell are (largely) removed from the coconut fat with the help of steam. If this process is carried out very gently and carefully, most of the nutrients (except for vitamin E) remain in the coconut fat.

If you want to be sure that it comprises all the health benefits that we are concerned with, you should buy only natural, virgin, and untreated coconut oil, preferably in raw quality, but under no circumstances refined or hydrogenated coconut fat, since the valuable substances are lost during these processes and trans fats are formed.

Coconut oil consists of 65 percent medium-chain fatty acids, also called MCTs (medium-chain triglycerides). These MCTs not only contain 10 percent fewer calories than long-chain saturated fatty acids (also known as LCTs, or long-chain triglycerides), but they are also easier to digest because they are transported directly from the intestine to the liver; other saturated fatty acids can be transported from the intestine to the liver only via the bloodstream. MCTs can also be absorbed and converted into energy more easily by the mitochondria. Because they are a faster source of energy than saturated fatty acids, they are not stored in fat deposits. As a supplement to the unsaturated fatty acids described below, coconut oil is the one saturated fat that should *not* be missing from the diet, but should always replace hydrogenated or refined fats.

Monounsaturated Fatty Acids

Like saturated fatty acids, our body can also produce a certain amount of monounsaturated fatty acids. But in order to have an adequate supply, we need to also ingest them through food, as they are responsible for the function and elasticity of our cell membranes, they lower the cholesterol level in the blood, and they prevent cardiovascular diseases. Monounsaturated fatty acids are predominantly found in plants, but also in fish and meat (beef), for example.

Olives, avocados, nuts, and oilseeds, such as pumpkin and sunflower seeds, linseed, sesame seeds, and poppy seeds, are all good sources of mono-unsaturated fatty acids. Monounsaturated fatty acids are abundant in many vegetable oils, such as rapeseed, olive, hemp, and linseed oil. When buying and consuming them, however, you should make sure that they are cold-pressed oils, as only cold pressing can preserve the flavors, vitamins, and mono- and polyunsaturated fatty acids.

More than 10 percent of our daily energy should be consumed from these in order to achieve a regulating and positive effect on the fat metabolism.

Polyunsaturated Fatty Acids

In contrast to saturated and monounsaturated fatty acids, the fatty acids in this group cannot be formed within our bodies. Since they are essential for life, they are also called essential fatty acids. They are a component of cell membranes, are involved in numerous metabolic processes, and, for example, keep the blood cholesterol level in balance. If we do not consume enough essential fatty acids, this can lead to deficiency symptoms and disorders such as hair loss, skin changes, susceptibility to infections, growth disorders, and depression, and in extreme cases also disorders of the immune system or impaired vision, concentration, and learning problems.

Pregnant women and breastfeeding mothers, but also children and people with preexisting illnesses and chronic inflammations, have a much greater need for polyunsaturated fatty acids, and science rightly attaches particular importance to them in the prevention of diabetes and many types of cancer. The essential fatty acids are divided into omega-3 fatty acids and omega-6 fatty acids, as already mentioned in connection with an anti-inflammatory diet.

Omega-3 Fatty Acids

Omega-3 fatty acids consist of alpha-linolenic acid (ALA), docosahexaenoic acid (DHA), and eicosapentaenoic acid (EPA); are found in abundance in certain (micro)algae; and are therefore predominantly found in cold-water fish such as herring, mackerel, tuna, sardines, and salmon, which feed on these algae.

Plant sources of omega-3 fatty acids are, for example, Brussels sprouts, spinach, beans, and avocados, as well as soy, nuts (especially walnuts), and seeds (mainly in linseed and Chia seeds). Cold-pressed and unheated oils of rapeseed, hemp, linseed, walnut, and Chia are also valuable sources of these essential fatty acids. Although plants, such as walnuts and linseed, contain significant amounts of omega-3 fatty acids, they are only converted to a limited extent into the active and important form of DHA in the organism. With a purely plant-based diet, it is therefore recommended to get your intake of healthy fats via a microalgae oil or a vegetable oil enriched with DHA and EPA.

The regular consumption of linseed oil nevertheless remains an important recommendation for everyone: Its positive effect on health, due to its high content of omega-3 and omega-6 fatty acids, has been researched in numerous studies. However, linseed oil is very sensitive to light and heat and therefore should be stored in a cool place away from light and not be heated.

Dr. Johanna Budwig's diet is all about the intake of these essential omega-3 fatty acids in the form of vegetable oils. According to her recommendations, it is above all linseed oil that, together with the sulfur-containing amino acids, forms the focus of her nutritional therapy. The essential fatty acid ALA, which is found in linseed oil or fish oils, improves—among other things—oxygen uptake in the mitochondria (see also section 3.9, "Mitochondria: Power Plants of the Cells," page 125). According to Budwig, a mixture of two tablespoons of linseed oil or fish oil with 200 grams of low-fat quark consumed daily improves oxygen utilization in our cells.

Omega-6 Fatty Acids

The most important fats of the omega-6 fatty acids are linoleic acid and the already mentioned arachidonic acid. Omega-6 fatty acids are not only a component of cell membranes, but are also needed for growth and repair processes. Linoleic acid, for example, is an important component of human skin and is partly responsible for regulating the water balance of the cells. In the case of skin damage, such as burns, linoleic acid is therefore also used externally. Sunflower, thistle, and walnut oils have a particularly high content of this fatty acid. Arachidonic acid helps the body produce tissue hormones that bring about inflammation as part of the immune defense. In a balanced, healthy immune system, this process is extremely helpful and important because inflammation can help the body to fight off dangerous pathogens in the case of infections.

Another effect of this fatty acid is an increased tendency of the blood to clot and a constriction of the blood vessels. The example of injuries shows how useful this can be; the faster the vessels constrict and the faster the blood platelets clump together, the less blood the body loses.

However, both examples make it clear that an excess of omega-3 acids can have negative effects: For one thing, an excess causes chronic inflammation, which weakens the body and creates the preconditions for further illnesses, such as cancer, rheumatism, and intestinal diseases, and for another thing, the risk of arteriosclerosis and thrombosis increases. A deficiency of omega-6 fatty acids is not possible with a balanced, nutritious diet, while at the same time an excess is avoided. In order to optimally support the body, a balanced ratio between the two fatty acids, omega-6 and omega-3, must be created: This ratio should be approximately at least 5:1.

Historically, a natural balance of the two essential fatty acids existed until industrialization. It is only since this time, and particularly since the end of the World War II, that our eating habits have changed in such a way that there is now a clear surplus of omega-6 fatty acids in our diets. This surplus of omega-6 fatty acids is caused by (too) high an intake of processed foods. At the same time, we do not consume enough omega-3 fatty acids. The average person in Western industrialized countries today consumes up to fifteen times more omega-6 fatty acids than omega-3 fatty acids, while young people consume up to twenty-five times more omega-6 acids. A change in the way we think and a health-conscious upbringing are urgently needed here—just as in other areas of nutrition—as with age it becomes more and more difficult to gain new insight and to change habits and behaviors.

3.2.6 The Healthy Microbiome: The Gut and Its Microorganisms

The gut microorganisms, also called the microbiome, consist of both the sum of the beneficial bacteria as well as the harmful bacteria and fungi that live in the gut. If the beneficial bacteria are predominant, we speak of a "healthy" or "balanced gut flora." However, if the harmful microorganisms can feed and multiply particularly well due to stress, bad diet, or taking medication (e.g., antibiotics), we speak of "disturbed gut flora."

To maintain a healthy gut flora or to correct an imbalance, a *dysbiosis*, we are advised to eat the foods mentioned above. In addition, our "good" gut bacteria feed predominantly and preferably on the high-fiber foods listed below.

Dietary Fibers

Vegetables and fruits (eaten with peel), dried fruits, whole-grain products, nuts (unsalted and not roasted), pulses, and seeds, including psyllium and linseed in particular, are valuable dietary fibers. Originally considered an "undesirable burden" (hence the German name "Ballaststoffe," literally translated as "burdensome substances") for the human digestive system, it is now clear how important these dietary fibers are for a healthy gut flora. As supportive and structural substances in the form of cellulose, hemicellulose, lignin, or pectin, they are just as important for plants as for our gut health.

A distinction is made between water-soluble and water-insoluble dietary fibers. Water-insoluble dietary fibers include cellulose, hemicellulose, and lignins, for example. Although they swell in water, they cannot be broken down by the intestinal bacteria, or if they are it is only to a small extent.

The water-soluble dietary fibers, such as pectin, form a gel-like substance when combined with water. They can be broken down, by intestinal bacteria in the large intestine, to carbon dioxide and other gases as well as to various short-chain fatty acids, which serve as nutrients for the cells of the intestinal mucosa. With their help, an acidic intestinal environment is maintained, which can optimally ward off pathogens. Because the valuable substances are mainly found in the cell walls and peels, it is always advisable to eat the peels of fruits and vegetables and to generally choose whole-grain products. The name "whole grain" comes from the fact that with these types of grain, the whole grain, including the shells and husks, too, is processed or milled.

For example, eating an orange with all its pith in between the segments is much healthier than drinking a glass of orange juice for this reason. The juice also has a lower vitamin and nutrient content while also having a higher sugar content than the whole orange.

————

In order for dietary fibers to swell sufficiently in the intestines, it is important to drink enough (mineral) water or unsweetened fruit or herbal teas. The recommendation is 1.5 liters a day.

As already explained in section 3.2.2 ("Detoxifying Substances in Food," page 46), fiber-rich food stimulates intestinal movements and delays gastric emptying to a healthy extent due to the lively activity, which also results in a prolonged feeling of satiety. The metabolism is regulated and the immune system is strengthened. Dietary fiber can also be taken as a food supplement, for example, in the form of psyllium or acacia fiber, to promote the detoxification of the body. We recommend a three-week course of intestinal cleansing powder at least once a year.

Potatoes Boiled in Their Skins

Since the potato has not yet received any honorable mention in our nutrition section, we would like to briefly introduce it here. Potatoes boiled in their skins are particularly friendly and helpful for intestinal bacteria. After boiling the potatoes, a gastric-acid-resistant starch is formed during cooling, which is broken down to butyric acid. This short-chain fatty acid serves as food for the epithelial cells of the intestines and provides them with energy. You can also keep a cooked supply in the fridge and treat yourself to a few boiled potatoes every now and then to do your intestinal cells some good. However, frying them to make fried potatoes is not advisable.

In Jairam K. P. Vanamala's research group in the Pennsylvania State College of Agricultural Sciences, the purple potato was specifically investigated with regard to colorectal cancer. The purple potato probably contains several substances that contribute to attacking or destroying cancer cells in the intestine through various mechanisms. In addition to the resistant starch, anthocyanins and chlorogenic acid are said to stimulate not only the ordinary cancer cells but also the cancer stem cells to self-destruct.

Researchers see a link to other fruits and vegetables in bright colors, as these brightly colored varieties contain, among other things, antioxidants that neutralize aggressive oxygen molecules in the body and thus have a particularly protective effect on the organism.

Lactic Acid Bacteria

In order to supply the lactic acid bacteria in the intestines, lactic acid fermented foods such as sauerkraut (also sauerkraut juice), kimchi, all lactic acid fermented vegetables, buttermilk, kefir, or yogurt should be consumed.

As long as these foods have not been heated to make them pasteurized—and thus, unfortunately, free of lactic acid bacteria—they contain the lactic acid bacteria that are important for the intestine. When buying foods that are advertised as *probiotic*, make sure that they do not contain added sugar.

Probiotics from the pharmacy are a better alternative for a targeted rebuilding of the intestinal flora. At least ten strains of bacteria should be contained in such a probiotic, as the many different types of bacteria in the intestine have different "nutritional preferences." Not least, the basis for healthy intestinal flora is stress-free eating.

3.2.7 Stress-Free Eating

Good eating habits are not only part of our intestinal health, but also the basis of the health of our entire organism.

Time

Meals should not be eaten in between doing other things and while standing or walking, but should be given the time they deserve. Rushing and stress when eating can, in the truest sense of the word, upset the stomach: A calm atmosphere, so that our senses can concentrate on the food, and enough time are important prerequisites so that we can eat our food without stress and then digest it well. Rushed gobbling down, eating food that is too hot, or perpetually eating a cold snack because you have to get going again in a hurry all put unnecessary strain on the stomach and intestines and lead to digestive problems such as abdominal pain, constipation, and flatulence.

With the help of saliva, the flow of which is stimulated by extensive chewing, the digestion of food begins in the mouth. Here, the food is prepared by certain enzymes that break down carbohydrates, in order to be further broken down into its components in the stomach with the support of gastric acid. If we regularly rush to eat and do not chew sufficiently, not only do our stomach and intestines have problems breaking down the food, but also we do not notice when we are actually full. The familiar feeling of fullness after a meal is not exclusively related to the amount of food eaten, but often also to the time it took to eat it: It takes about twenty minutes for the stomach to signal to the brain whether enough food has been consumed.

People who often eat quickly until they "can't manage any more" also put a strain on their whole organism. The regular *excess* thus often translates to gained weight.

For this reason, in Japan there is said to be a behavior of always finishing a meal before feeling full, which is estimated to correspond to only 70 percent of a meal. Since the stomach *lags behind* a little with its reporting, as just mentioned, this method can be used to determine after a while that 70 percent is enough to feel sufficiently full.

Disruptive Factors

In our busy and multimedia (Western) world, we are now subject to constant noise, ringing, and chatter, and there are more and more moving images (with sound) on flatscreens, even in restaurants, bars, and cafes.

Above all, we should have a break from the phone, computer, and television, but also the radio, a book, or a newspaper when we're eating, so that we can concentrate fully on the food. Our senses are otherwise occupied with absorbing and processing the information and not with absorbing and processing the food.

Appreciation and Regularity

A fresh, diverse, and varied diet is also associated with a certain self-worth. Only those who value themselves will allow themselves the regular preparation of good food. Valuing yourself, the perception of your own and actual needs, is a prerequisite for a fulfilled, healthy life. A positive attitude toward life, respect for yourself and other living beings, one could even say a true or real self-love, leads to doing good for yourself and others. The proverb "the way to a man's heart is through his stomach" is often used with a smile to describe lovers cooking together, but it actually shows quite well how we relate to ourselves and our world/surroundings. The regularity of our meals or whether we want to eat anything at all can also reflect this to a certain extent. Apart from the already mentioned intermittent fasting, a (regular) fasting day or a fasting cure, it is not healthy to (consciously) starve yourself again and again. Depending on the exertion and strain on our organism, we should meet the need to eat sufficient and healthy food and eat regularly in a way that allows our body to function as well as possible.

Rest Breaks

On the other hand, in the case of a lack of energy, it may also be appropriate to help the organism regain energy not by eating but, for example, by getting enough sleep and taking regular breaks for sleep and rest. The body can also signal a desire for food when the underlying need is actually relaxation or sleep, or when we should be attending to our body (and mind) in other ways.

The Exception Proves the Rule

Since we all deal differently with rules and their deployment and adherence, stress-free eating or stress-free eating habits ultimately include the exception: Unless we are supposed to stick to a strict diet plan for a certain period of time for medical reasons, a glass of wine, dark chocolate, or similar treats should not lead to a bad conscience or unnecessary stress. If you want to eat a vegetarian or vegan diet for ethical reasons, you should pay close attention to plant-based fats and oils, proteins, and minerals. Otherwise, eating good-quality meat or fish raised with species-appropriate husbandry presents a healthy exception to the vegetarian diverse and fresh diet.

If we generally eat a varied, diverse, and fresh diet, it is not a problem if one (unhealthy) exception proves the rule.

3.2.8 A Diet That Lowers Blood Glucose Levels

It is advisable—not only in the case of diabetes, but also more generally—to establish a stable blood glucose level with little fluctuation. The diet that should keep blood sugar at a constant level as much as possible is called the low-carb diet, which is significantly reduced in carbohydrates. At the same time, however, this diet should be clearly distinguished from the ketogenic diet.

In the low-carb diet, the carbohydrate content should only be 15–30 percent of the daily intake, or twenty to eighty grams per day. It is important that the carbohydrates we eat have a low glycemic index. The glycemic index is a measure of the effect of food on blood sugar level, or how quickly a nutrient is converted into sugar in our organism (more on this in chapter 6).

It is well known by now that, in general, only small amounts of sugar and sugar substitutes should be consumed, and too much sweet and processed food should be avoided for health reasons. The situation is more complex when it comes to carbohydrates. The *good* carbohydrates, such as whole-grain products and legumes, have already been mentioned several times and will be mentioned again and again in the following. They may and should be part of our daily menu, even when following a low-carb diet.

Legumes

Legumes, for example, are digested more slowly than potatoes, rice, or pasta. However—as already mentioned—brown rice or whole-grain pasta is significantly different from white rice or pasta made from durum wheat: Blood glucose level rises less quickly (relatively low glycemic index) with pulses and whole-grain products, a feeling of satiety is maintained for longer, and there are none of the extreme hunger pangs that are the result of a rapidly rising and then rapidly falling blood glucose level. Protein-rich peas and lentils in particular stimulate the production of short-chain fatty acids, which can lower an already existing increase in blood glucose level.

Oily Fish

Fresh, oily fish such as salmon, herring, sardines, and mackerel, as well as lean fish such as trout and cod, only raise blood sugar moderately, and the high protein content and amino acids they contain ensure that the feeling of satiety lasts longer after a meal containing oily fish. The omega-3 fatty acids in oily fish are protective against heart attacks and strokes, as DHA and EPA keep the heart and arteries healthy.

Green Leafy Vegetables

Green leafy vegetables also provide the body with only very small amounts of sugar. Due to the hard-to-digest plant fibers (already mentioned under dietary fibers), green leafy vegetables are particularly filling for a long time and contain few calories and carbohydrates. This helps to keep blood sugar levels constant. Green leafy vegetables also support healthy glucose levels and can be used in almost any form for green smoothies.

Healthy Fats

Good fats have also already been mentioned. They slow down the release of glucose in the intestine and can be added to the meal in the form of various oils (especially virgin olive oil, but also rapeseed, sunflower, sesame, walnut, pumpkin, safflower, soybean, or peanut oil). They contain the blood-sugar-regulating mono- or polyunsaturated fatty acids. Avocados, nuts, olives, and pumpkin, sunflower, and other seeds also provide valuable fats that lower blood sugar and can be eaten as a snack between meals. When consuming olive oil, you should only use extra virgin oil, which can lower harmful LDL cholesterol levels as well as blood sugar.

Garlic

Just like virgin olive oil, garlic has positive effects on blood sugar levels and reduces the proportion of bad LDL cholesterol in blood fats.

Cinnamon

This tasty spice slows down the breakdown of carbohydrates in the digestive tract and thus reduces the increase in blood sugar after a meal. Cinnamon acts like insulin, but more slowly, and slows down the glucose reaction. A daily dose of one to six grams (half a teaspoon to two level teaspoons) is an effective, health-promoting amount, but this should not be exceeded. You should use cinnamon not only at Christmastime, but also in daily smoothies, in Indian-style cuisine, and in yogurt and fruit dishes.

Cocoa

Dark chocolate with a minimum cocoa content of 85 percent contains not only much less added sugar but also more of the polyphenols epicatechin and catechin. With these polyphenols' help, dark chocolate also alters the glucose metabolism in the intestine and stimulates insulin production in the pancreas. This helps the body to react better to high blood sugar levels.

Regular cocoa consumption is said to have a greater effect on insulin resistance than single doses of cocoa products. Here, it is also important to look for good quality and as little added sugar as possible. This means that chocolate consumption should be limited to one or two pieces of dark chocolate per day, and if you drink hot chocolate, you should make it yourself from cocoa powder, adding only a little (raw cane) sugar or honey. This only works with warm or hot cow, rice, oat, almond, soy, or coconut milk in order to dissolve the fat. Once the tastebuds have become accustomed to it, chocolate with a high cocoa percentage or only slightly sweetened cocoa is the purest indulgence that also tastes like real cocoa.

Cider Vinegar

The acetic acid of fruit vinegar can slow down the digestion of glucose and thus reduce the rise in blood sugar level after eating. The organism has more time to metabolize the sugar in the blood, and rapidly rising sugar spikes can be prevented. The greater the acidity of vinegar, the more effectively it can lower the blood sugar and insulin response after a meal. Vinegar is also said to increase the subjective feeling of satiety. Cider vinegar can be added to salad dressings or drunk after a meal, mixed with a glass of water. However, if you are taking diabetes medication at the same time, you should check with your doctor whether the effect of the vinegar is compatible with other medications you are taking. For simple refreshment or to boost the metabolism in the morning, a fruit vinegar lemonade is something which has been popular since ancient times.

Fruit vinegar can also be used to lose weight in slimming diets. For this reason, this otherwise refreshing and healthy drink is not suitable for people who are already underweight or who suffer from tumor cachexia (consumption or emaciation in cancer patients) and should not be consumed in this case.

Food Supplements for a Balanced Insulin Level

As a natural remedy, berberine (alkaloid from barberry) is known for its blood-sugar-regulating properties. Berberine activates an enzyme in our tissues that improves sensitivity to insulin, thereby counteracting blood sugar spikes and an excess of insulin production. Berberine is becoming increasingly popular for facilitating weight loss, lowering blood cholesterol levels, and improving blood sugar regulation.

Among the micronutrients, chromium plays an important role in regulating blood sugar levels and is a common deficiency for humans. Taking an organic chromium salt, chromium picolinate, can improve blood sugar regulation and also fat metabolism.

3.2.9 A Diet That Strengthens the Immune System

The varied, fresh, mixed diet discussed here is a diet that optimally supports the immune system. The balance of the diet is also an important prerequisite for an intact immune system from the point of view of defense. For these defense mechanisms to function optimally, vitamins and minerals must be available to the organism in sufficient quantities. The previously mentioned fats, dietary fibers, and secondary plant substances also play an important role.

However, the function of the immune system can also be influenced by body weight, and an increased susceptibility to infections can thus be brought about by being underweight as well as overweight. Everything that has been mentioned so far as being anti-inflammatory, detoxifying, oxygen-enriching, beneficial to intestinal health, and so forth, also contributes to strengthening the immune system and the last three vital fields. As already mentioned elsewhere, secondary plant substances and probiotic foods are extremely important for strengthening the immune system. Therefore, we now turn to individual vitamins and minerals as food supplements.

Food Supplements for a Strong Immune System

VITAMIN C

The advice to take vitamin C when suffering from infections is well known. In high doses, it can not only boost the immune system in stressful situations, for example, by supporting the white blood cells that are needed and used up en masse during infections, but it is also frequently and successfully used in cancer therapy. For an optimally strengthened immune system, at least five hundred to one thousand milligrams of vitamin C should be taken daily. The consumption of citrus fruits or berries containing vitamin C, especially the acerola cherry, is the most natural way to take vitamin C in a biologically high-quality form. However, it is hardly possible to consume therapeutically high amounts of vitamin C in the gram range in the form of natural vitamin C. In stressful situations, it is therefore recommended to take food supplements with a high vitamin C content. For the anticancer effect of very high doses of vitamin C (thirty to one hundred grams) in the form of an infusion, see chapter 6. Dietary supplements in capsule form using natural sources of vitamin C, such as acerola cherries, sea buckthorn, rosehips, currants, strawberries, papaya, citrus fruits, kiwi, Braeburn apples or red pepper, broccoli, cabbage, fresh green herbs, and green beans, reach dosages of over one hundred micrograms of bioavailable Vitamin C per capsule.

Higher doses of oral vitamin C (up to several grams per serving) can be obtained by taking pure vitamin C powder (usually made from starch). Mixed with water, it is best taken in a pH-neutral form, for example, as sodium ascorbate or magnesium ascorbate, which does not damage the stomach lining by the acid effect of pure ascorbic acid.

PRO VITAMIN D_3

This vitamin is strictly speaking not a real vitamin, but rather is a hormone precursor. The body can produce prohormone vitamin D_3 itself with sufficient exposure to sunlight, and only a small amount is absorbed through food. However, the body's own production, the given circumstances in our latitudes, and the supply via food are not sufficient in most cases, so most people have a vitamin D deficiency, and this deficiency is more widespread than is generally claimed. The fat-soluble prohormone vitamin D_3, also called cholecalciferol, promotes the formation and maturation of bone stem cells, regulates the mineralization of bones, and strengthens muscles. For some years now, however, it has become increasingly clear that it is also necessary for a strong and balanced immune system; has a positive effect on the psyche, the cardiovascular system, and vascular diseases; and has a protective effect for the nerve cells in the brain and against cancer (cells).

Almost all cells in our body need vitamin D for the optimal control of their intracellular processes, which is why it also fulfils countless purposes in the body. The diversity of its purposes simultaneously shows that a lack of vitamin D can lead to the widest variety of health problems.

We can get some vitamin D from fatty fish (including cod liver oil or fish oil), eggs, or veal liver. Avocados also contain some vitamin D, but vegetarians and vegans are strongly advised to take supplements. Vitamin D, ideally combined with vitamin K_2, is increasingly recommended by doctors, therapists, and alternative practitioners and should be taken by people living in the northern hemisphere, at least in the sunshine-lacking months between October and March.

B VITAMINS

A deficiency of B vitamins can also weaken the immune system and promote numerous diseases (such as dementia). Vitamins B_6, B_{12}, and B_9 (also known as folic acid or folate) have been shown to have a direct positive effect on the immune system. They are found in potatoes, bananas, legumes, spinach, lamb's lettuce, cabbage, nuts, seeds, and animal liver. We can meet our need for vitamin B_{12} exclusively through animal products such as fish, meat, eggs, and dairy products. Vegans are strongly advised to take a supplement, and possibly even those of us who eat only small amounts of animal products. Similar to vitamin D deficiency, vitamin B_{12} deficiency also manifests itself in chronic fatigue, forgetfulness, and depressive moods.

IRON AND ZINC

Iron is the most common trace element and, like zinc, which is the second most common trace element; iron is very important for our organism. An adult needs between ten milligrams (men) and fifteen grams (menstruating women) of iron per day. It is responsible for the formation of red blood cells and the transport of oxygen in the blood and is a component of many enzymes. The immune system cannot function optimally in the case of iron deficiency, and disorders manifest themselves in infections and inflammations, fatigue and listlessness, skin and mucous membrane diseases, and even hair loss.

Chronic diseases can in turn lead to iron deficiency, but also blood loss or advancing age. Women, vegetarians, and vegans can be particularly affected by this deficiency and should take iron supplements if they have been diagnosed as deficient by a doctor.

Vitamin C promotes the absorption of iron as well as of zinc. The bioavailability of zinc is also improved by animal protein.

The body's zinc storage is very low and therefore zinc must be supplied sufficiently through food or dietary supplements. Large parts of the immune system are limited in their function if there is a zinc deficiency: An increased likelihood of inflammation is the result if, for example, macrophages (scavenger cells), granulocytes, natural killer cells, T cells, and B cells are not sufficiently supplied with zinc. But also zinc deficiency can result in various diseases, from infections and allergies to strokes, Alzheimer's, depression, and even arteriosclerosis, diabetes, and cancer.

Although the ratio of absorption-promoting and absorption-inhibiting food ingredients is quite complex in the case of zinc and iron, it is naturally balanced in the varied, colorful, low-carbohydrate, and oily and nutty Mediterranean mixed diet that we recommend here in this book. An individual, additional need should be checked by your doctor through blood tests and, if necessary, remedied through the administration of dietary supplements.

SELENIUM

Selenium also has enormous importance for our immune defense and serves as a protection against chronic inflammation and cancers. Selenium is involved in all those enzyme systems that fight free radicals in the body and is therefore indirectly responsible for the optimal functioning of these enzymes and the defense reactions associated with them. Oxidative stress can lead to malignant tumor growth, which is why a sufficient and if necessary additional selenium intake is key to support of the antioxidant defense system. Meanwhile, it has been proven that patients with cancerous tumors generally have a selenium level that is too low.

In the northern latitudes, it is almost impossible to get sufficient amounts of this trace element through our food: A significant selenium content can only be found in legumes and asparagus. Additional sources of selenium in northern Europe are meat, fish, yeast, and eggs, but they are far from sufficient. The intake of selenium, which goes beyond a mere deficiency precaution, should be one hundred to three hundred micrograms per day, which is possible in countries such as Japan, Canada, or Venezuela due to the soil conditions.

Selenium should not be taken together with vitamin C, as the effect of both substances is weakened when taken in one capsule or at the same time.

3.2.10 A Diet That Strengthens the Mitochondria

The intake of vital substances through fresh and varied fruits and vegetables, the supply of healthy fats through vegetable oils, but also through dairy products and fish, "embedded" in a diet rich in fiber, is already the diet that ensures an optimal supply of energy and oxygen to the mitochondria.

Chapter 2 "illuminates" how vital substances have a direct relationship to our cellular power plants and what positive effects they have when we

consume them—as described—through a healthy diet and the corresponding dietary supplements with their twelve vital fields.

But we can also see a direct connection between section 3.9, "Mitochondria:
Power Plants of the Cells" (page 125) and section 3.1, "The Detoxification of
the Organism" (page 32) and even this section, and we can notice an immediate and beneficial effect, for example, with the anti-inflammatory diet or
the intake of good carbohydrates. The already mentioned Budwig diet also
supports the energy supply of the mitochondria in a certain way.

Green smoothies (one way of supplying vital substances), saturated
fatty acids, and certain food supplements such as selenium, L-carnitine,
acetylcysteine, zinc, and magnesium, as well as intermittent fasting as a
mitochondrial-strengthening measure, have a particularly positive effect on
the function of our mitochondria. Intermittent fasting has been intensively
researched, especially by the Italian-American gerontologist Valter Longo.

Longo describes in detail the benefits that the healthy starvation of intermittent fasting can have, as long as you have a good perception of your own
body and how it should be performing and do not exceed its limits.

As also mentioned elsewhere in this book, our bodies are actually designed
to eat less rich food than is the case in our Western way of life today. From
this perspective, intermittent fasting is certainly not harmful.

However, in the case of specific cancers or at a certain stage of cancer
and the possible associated emaciation, good or deliberate starvation may no
longer have any benefits but will have the opposite effect. In such cases, it is
particularly important not to try any other forms of dieting or—for whatever
reason—to forgo certain things, as this would only further weaken the organism and advance cachexia (emaciation with a BMI of less than 18 kg/m²). In
addition to the unsaturated fatty acids described above, saturated fatty acids
such as coconut oil or coconut puree, which contain a high proportion of
lauric acid, are of particular importance.

Lauric acid belongs to the MCTs. They provide the body with energy
quickly and relatively easily. MCTs are therefore just what the mitochondria
need. In the body, lauric acid acts against viruses, microbes, (yeast) fungi, and
bacteria and is antimicrobial as well as antibacterial, in that it can destroy the
outer membrane of lipids in the cases of viruses, for example, and the virus
perishes as a result of the released interior.

Coconut oil and coconut puree can be used as the basis of the fat supply, supplemented by butter and ghee (cooked, milk-protein-free clarified butter), which are also well suited for cooking, as they do not oxidize at high heats the way vegetable oils do.

The intake of vital substances can be particularly supported by consuming the aforementioned smoothies, in particular green smoothies.

The case for green smoothies is rooted in the fact that abundant chlorophyll contained in leaves is responsible for photosynthesis in plants. The green chlorophyll transforms sunlight during photosynthesis into micronutrients such as vitamins, minerals, trace elements, and so forth, that are valuable to our organism. Just like the cells of plants, the mitochondria of our cells need these micronutrients for metabolism.

A high-performance blender suitable for the preparation of smoothies with a speed of twenty-five thousand revolutions or more per minute crushes green leafy vegetables and herbs much more thoroughly than we can achieve even with extensive chewing, and makes the plant micronutrients available to our organism in an optimal way.

Green smoothies should be consumed on an empty stomach. They are to be considered like a meal—including chewing—and can be enjoyed until a feeling of satiety sets in. They should be half green leaves and half fruit. If dried fruit is being pureed, correspondingly less is needed than in the case of fresh fruit. The entire contents are pureed with fresh, filtered and/or revitalized water to form a creamy, thick mass.

Here, too, we can take our cue from nature's seasonal and regional diversity and use those leafy vegetables and wild herbs that are growing at the moment and have traveled as short a distance as possible.

If you're looking for a more precise recipe for making green or other healthy smoothies, you can find various recipes on the internet or in many different books.

Dietary Supplements for Healthy Mitochondria

To support mitochondrial function and, if necessary, to treat mitochondrial diseases or weaknesses, a number of natural substances are available that we can ingest via our food or special dietary supplements. The biochemistry of these substances in our mitochondria is the subject of countless books and is constantly being researched further. The most important substances for improving mitochondrial activity are briefly mentioned and described here.

D-RIBOSE

D-ribose is a simple sugar molecule with five carbon atoms and provides quickly accessible energy especially to the heart and brain cells, which are among the most mitochondria-rich cells in our body, with several thousand mitochondria per cell. Stirred into water by the teaspoonful, it can bring about a rapid energy improvement in our mitochondria.

COQ10

CoQ10 (coenzyme Q10) and PQQ (pyrroloquinoline quinone) are other extensively researched naturally occurring substances used for mitochondrial strengthening.

MAGNESIUM

Magnesium is one of the most underestimated minerals that we need every day. There are many reasons in our modern lifestyle that explain why only a few people (an estimated 20–30 percent) have an optimal magnesium level in their body, for example, too much calcium intake from food, decalcifiers that bind magnesium from water, medications for heartburn, and high coffee consumption. Magnesium is the cofactor for over three hundred biochemical reactions in our organism, including the production of energy in our mitochondria.

ALPHA LIPOIC ACID

Alpha lipoic acid, creatine, B vitamins, resveratrol—found mainly in grapes and red wine—and pterostilbene—found, for example, in blueberries, but also in grapes and the padouk, a tree from tropical West Africa—are other natural substances that support our mitochondria.

KETOGENIC DIET

The ketogenic diet—with a carbohydrate content of less than fifty grams per day—or even calorie restriction (fasting), has the effect of, among other things, activating the mitochondria.

L-CARNITINE

L-carnitine plays a particular role for the mitochondria. Our mitochondria need fats to produce the ATP (adenosine triphosphate) from ADP (adenosine diphosphate) that is needed everywhere in the organism. However, L-carnitine is needed so that fats can pass through the mitochondrial membrane. L-carnitine is chemically an ammonium compound and is produced in our cells from the amino acids lysine and methionine. It can also be taken as a dietary supplement. Doses of two to three grams per day, for example, can stimulate fat metabolism in our mitochondria, which improves the energy supply to brain cells, mood, and performance, and results in greater resistance to stress.

The book *Mitochondria and the Future of Medicine* by Lee Know describes the current state of knowledge regarding the biochemistry of mitochondria. If you want to find out more, you can find further interesting, detailed information there.

3.2.11 A Diet That Maintains the Acid–Base Balance

Chemical processes are constantly taking place in our body so that our metabolism can function, so that we can control our muscles, and so that stimuli can be transmitted.

The basis for a smooth process is a maintained acid–base balance. It is expressed as the pH value by determining the concentration of hydrogen ions in a liquid. By definition, the physiological pH of the human organism is in the range of 7.35 to 7.45. However, with our current lifestyle and diet, the pH of our tissues is often disturbed or out of balance. A diet with too much meat and other protein-containing foods and dairy products from conventional production, white flour products, sugar, caffeinated and carbonated drinks, convenience foods and canned foods, alcohol, and stress, but not enough vegetables, fruits, and fluids, as well as a lack of relaxation and physical exercise, can lead to a chronic acidification in the organism and to acute or chronic diseases. Inflammations or an unbalanced intestinal flora can also negatively influence the acid–base balance.

With an acid-forming diet and lifestyle, sulfuric acid and other harmful substances are produced in the body, which are generally also referred to

Table 3.1. Base-forming Fruits

Berries	Blueberries, blackberries, strawberries, bilberries, raspberries, red currants, cranberries, gooseberries
Pome fruits	Apples, pears, medlars, quince
Nuts	Almonds, tiger nuts, sweet chestnuts, macadamia, Brazil nuts, fresh walnuts
Stone fruits	Apricots, cherries, mirabelle plums, nectarines, olives, peaches, plums, greengages, damsons
Southern fruits	Pineapples, bananas, dates, figs, kiwis, mangos, papayas, star fruits, grapes
Citrus fruits	Clementines, grapefruit, limes, mandarins, oranges, lemons

as waste products. These are toxins that the organism normally eliminates from the body with its detoxifying organs and mechanisms. But a constant imbalance cannot be sufficiently balanced. Because hyperacidity usually develops slowly over many years, symptoms tend to be rather unspecific, but can manifest themselves in a weakened immune system and a damaged intestinal flora and occur, for example, in the form of circulatory disorders, neurodermatitis, metabolic disorders, stomach problems, gout, or rheumatism. An alkaline diet supports the body's detoxification organs and prevents an environment that favors diseases.

Foods are therefore also classified as acid forming or base forming. Only a quarter of the daily diet should consist of acid-forming foods in order to not overload the organism. Base foods are characterized by base-forming minerals and trace elements and have plenty of iron, magnesium, potassium, and calcium, numerous vitamins, antioxidants, and secondary plant substances that support the body's own formation of bases. The bases in turn help the organism to eliminate acids and toxins. The majority of fruits and vegetables are base forming, as are vegetable fats and oils. As a sweetener, honey is a good base-former. Among drinks, herbal teas, still water, and smoothies (especially green smoothies) are base forming.

Table 3.2. Base-forming Vegetables

Leafy vegetables	Lettuce, oakleaf lettuce, iceberg lettuce, lamb's lettuce, Lollo lettuce, rocket, radicchio, chicory and dandelion, chard, spinach, celery, purslane and Chinese cabbage, kale, kohlrabi, pak choi, Brussels sprouts, red cabbage, pointed cabbage, white cabbage, savoy cabbage
Flowering vegetables	Artichokes, cauliflower, broccoli, romanesco
Fruit vegetables	Aubergines, avocados, cucumbers, pumpkins, melons, okra, peppers, tomatoes, courgettes, avocados
Tubers and root vegetables	Fennel, carrots, beetroot, horseradish, radishes, potatoes, parsnips, parsley root, celeriac, sweet potatoes, black salsify
Seed vegetables	Beans, green beans, peas, mung beans, lentils, and soya bean sprouts
Vegetables in the onion family	Leeks, cress, garlic, shallots, chives, onions
Herbs	Basil, savory, nettles, dill, chervil, coriander, lovage, marjoram, parsley, peppermint, oregano, rosemary, sage, sorrel, chives, thyme, wild herbs, lemon balm
Mushrooms	Oyster mushrooms, button mushrooms, wood ear mushrooms, shiitake mushrooms, porcini mushrooms, truffle mushrooms
Spices	Chili pepper, ginger, cumin, caraway, turmeric, nutmeg, cloves, pepper, allspice, saffron, vanilla, cinnamon
Sprouts	Alfalfa, brown millet and millet sprouts, wheat, spelt and barley sprouts, mung bean, lentil and soybean sprouts

In a healthy diet, which should keep acids and bases in balance, a further distinction is made between good-acid-forming foods and bad-acid-forming foods. The good-acid-forming foods can and should be a regular part of the diet, the bad ones—as explained at the beginning of this chapter—should be consumed rarely or not at all.

Legumes are good acid-formers, as are oats and oat flakes, millet and whole-grain rice, oilseeds—for example, sunflower seeds, pumpkin seeds, sesame seeds, poppy seeds, or linseed—pseudocereals—for example, quinoa, amaranth, and buckwheat—tofu, and high-quality fermented soy products such as miso and tempeh.

For drinks, good acid-formers include green tea and matcha, high-quality plant-based (milk substitute) drinks, such as rice drink, oat drink, and soy drink, of course all without sweeteners, flavorings, and thickeners, as well as homemade drinking chocolate made from pure, high-quality cocoa powder. Coffee in moderation, drunk as espresso and not as filter coffee, also has a slightly alkaline effect. Organic eggs and organic fish are also recommended in moderation.

With regard to the base-forming properties of foodstuffs, it makes sense to select only high-quality, organic foods, as they have a higher content of minerals and trace elements that have an alkaline-positive effect.

Due to conventional cultivation, fruits, vegetables, and grains are usually loaded with herbicides, pesticides, heavy metals, nitrate, and phosphate, which overload the organism. As explained at the beginning of the chapter, this can lead to gradual hyperacidity.

Sports and physical exercise, along with a balanced, alkaline diet, are important for the acid–base balance, as the metabolism is stimulated and acids are excreted via the kidneys, lungs, and skin. Other detoxifying measures, such as alkaline partial baths, brush massages, saunas, and so forth, are also beneficial.

If your body is already overacidic, you can also take an alkaline powder to help regulate the imbalance, but it cannot replace the consumption of base-forming foods.

The Base-forming Fruits and Base-forming Vegetables tables offer some examples of base-forming fruits and (fresh) vegetables, subdivided according to use. Dried fruits are also base-forming.

3.2.12 Nutrition for a Strong Defense against Infections

Having arrived at the last vital field, nutrition for a strong defense against infections, there really is nothing essential to add to what has been said so far with regard to nutrition. Our assumption that everything is interrelated is once again supported by this. The organism is best prepared for a successful defense against infections if the recommendations of the eleven fields can be partially or completely integrated and implemented in normal everyday life.

The overall picture shows that intestinal health is closely linked to an anti-inflammatory diet. This, in turn, consists of a balanced, nutrient-rich diet that supplies the organism and its cells with sufficient oxygen, has an insulin-regulating effect, and also keeps the body's acid–base balance in equilibrium, as well as supplying the mitochondria, protecting the immune system, and strengthening the defense against infections.

This back-and-forth of influencing factors could be continued endlessly.

The fact that a lot is repeated, overlapped, or complemented in the previous sections is a sign of the coherence of the various assertions and ultimately is a blessing for us, as there is no need for great promises of salvation in the form of extreme diets, behavioral changes, or ever-new product applications. What we are, how we eat, behave, and deal with our body is the basis for giving ourselves the optimal care within this systemic structure.

This twelfth vital field is therefore meant to be the final plea that any field can be complemented by or related to any other. Using the image of a mobile, this means that we initially have to only trigger one or two fields in order to perceive a movement in the overall structure, to perceive a change or improvement.

However, particularly in the area of nutrition and the associated effect on our organism, it is, of course, not so easy to recognize or localize which behavior, which diets, and which foods trigger, improve, support, or prevent exactly this or that. Where a rash has come from may not be as immediately clear as how we can track the movement of a mobile. What is certain, however, is that the holistic system is in a relationship with itself in every conceivable way and that there are lots of connections that work for us.

Here, too, the perspective is repeated: "The large scale reflects the small scale." The image of microcosm and macrocosm, in which every organism, no matter how small, is connected to a structure that goes beyond it, and this structure in turn has relationships to a larger complex system, can also illustrate here how both the cells of our organism and we as human beings, as well as our environment, are constantly related to each other and are in constant exchange with each other.

3.3 Water: An Elixir of Life

3.3.1 The Importance of Water for Body and Mind

Earth is the planet of water. Its inhabitants are beings flowed through by and dependent on water. Approximately 70 percent of the earth's surface is covered by water. It is remarkable that this also corresponds to the proportion of water by weight in the adult human body. If you calculate what percentage of all molecules in our bodies are made up of water, you arrive at the almost unbelievable figure of 99 percent. This is partly due to the fact that the H_2O molecule is small compared to most macromolecules in our body.

To keep our organism alive and healthy, we need between thirty-five and forty milliliters of water per kilogram of body weight per day. For an adult weighing seventy-five kilograms, this amounts to just under three liters.

Water is the universal life carrier not only in humans but in all life processes. Water transports all substances dissolved in it, in our cells, in the blood, and in the lymph. It gives structure to our proteins and many of the macromolecules that make up our bodies through hydrogen bonds. Also called Van der Waals forces, these electrical charges provide the bonds between all molecules of the living organism. Water enables all chemical reactions in our metabolism. And finally, thanks to water, we maintain our biochemical balances as long as we are healthy: the acid–base balance, our body heat, all metabolic balances, and what we refer to with the ancient Greek term *homeostasis*—the equilibrium or balance of the life-creating and life-sustaining forces.

Let's take a closer look at the smallest building block of water, the H_2O molecule. It is known to consist of one oxygen and two hydrogen atoms. What is of greatest importance here is that the electrical charges of this molecule are unequally, polarly distributed. Water is a polar molecule, with an electrically positive pole and an electrically negative pole. The larger oxygen atom (O atom) attracts the electrons of the smaller hydrogen atoms (H atoms) toward it. Since positive and negative poles attract each other, the result is that the water molecules attract one another. This leads to the fact that water consists of H_2O molecules that are more or less cross-linked with one another, forming clusters, groups, heaps, or agglomerations.

Water that is in motion naturally, for example, in a stream, or was just a moment ago, is made up of fewer interlocked water clusters, one could also say it is less or hardly *clumped together*. Water, on the other hand, that has been standing still for a long time—which is the case, for example, in our water pipes—consists of H_2O molecules clumped together in larger clusters.

Whether water has a fine, small-membered and very mobile cluster structure or its molecules are clumped together in large clusters has enormous significance for its properties in living organisms.

What at first sight may read like a physical subtlety is not only of the utmost importance for all living creatures on our planet, but also for the course of seasonal phenomena, such as from ice to cloud formations and meteorology.

The American biophysicist Gerald H. Pollack has researched these phenomena, which were unknown until a few years ago, and described them in his book *Water: Much More Than H_2O* in a way that is understandable even for interested nonphysicists.

He reports on a fourth state of aggregation of water, which it can assume in addition to the three known manifestations of gaseous, liquid, and solid—steam, water, and ice—when it is close to an interface, as is the case, for example, with proteins in our blood or the membranes of our body cells.

This water—like a liquid crystal—has a special *inner structure*, just like naturally occurring water from springs, rainwater, or fresh meltwater from glaciers, which is structured in the same way.

Professor Pollack therefore calls this water in its fourth state of aggregation EZ water, meaning "exclusion zone water." The *exclusion zone* is the region in the immediate vicinity of cell membranes that contains the most finely structured water, or EZ water, which is distinguished from normal water that contains larger cluster structures.

Water that is structured in this way promotes life processes better than water that has stood still for a long time—days to weeks—or has flowed in straightened pathways (pipes) and whose water molecules have clustered together.

The fine, mobile structure of EZ water can easily pass through the water channels of the cell walls, called aquaporins; in this way, the cells are always supplied with sufficient water. Structured water also helps the proteins in our body to form the correct structure (see also chapter 2), helps this correct structure to be absorbed and passed on to organisms and cells, and helps our bodies to eliminate toxins more effectively. It also promotes the optimal energy production in our mitochondria.

According to Pollack, EZ water has a great significance for our health. Diseases could be associated with our cells not getting enough EZ water because it is found in sufficient quantities only in pure, freshly bottled spring water. A lack of structured water may even play an important role in cancer development. In his book *Cells, Gels and the Engines of Life*, Pollack wrote that "anything that promotes water structure formation inhibits tumor growth. [. . .] Agents that promote water ordering are predicted to inhibit tumor proliferation. To my knowledge this approach has not yet been tested. Nor is it established whether the reputed efficacy of some anticancer agents might lie in such a mechanism."

A huge statement, the implications of which hardly anyone can guess at today. Could it be that unstructured, *clumped* or clustered water, which is now the rule for our drinking water and no longer the exception (who drinks fresh spring or glacier water?), is contributing to the development of more and more cancers around the world?

The water described here—in a state between solid and liquid—is more viscous, more alkaline, negatively charged, and also somewhat denser and more energetic than disordered water. In its structure, the water molecules resemble a honeycomb with a hexagonal shape and have the chemical formula H_3O_2. This structure is found not only on earth in hexagonal honeycombs and in volcanic basaltic rocks and the hexagonal form of snow crystals—as long as the water is undamaged and *healthy*—but also on the surface of the sun. See figure 3.1.

Is it pure coincidence that exactly these forms (and formulae) also appear in nature and even on the surface of the sun, or is a universal design principle expressed here? Researchers like

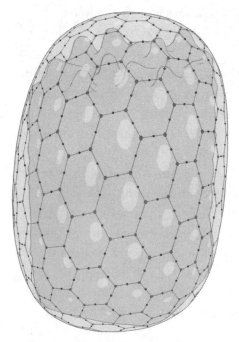

Figure 3.1. Cell with hexagonal H_2O shell.

Rupert Sheldrake speak of "morphogenetic fields," fields of force that create forms in the world of matter, a thoroughly interesting hypothesis, for which there are now many observations. Especially since the phenomenon of the forms of living creatures has not yet received a convincing explanation in a scientific way. It is simply accepted and not questioned further as to who or what actually formed the shapes of, for example, our liver or our heart. To refer to genes as an answer to this question misses the point and only shifts it to the level of smaller forms, without answering it. After half a lifetime as a doctor and vital researcher, to me, the assumption of a form-creating force field still seems the best answer. From a physical point of view, electromagnetic forces can be observed and measured everywhere in the universe. The countless phenomena of living creatures indicate that there are other, more subtle and as yet unmeasurable life forces "behind it." These need to be explored further. Traditional medical teachings have spoken for thousands of years about qi or prana as the universal life forces, for which there is still no physical measure. It therefore seems obvious to see the human being as an energy being, and in such a being, the water molecule plays a fundamental and decisive role for our health.

3.3.2 The Treatment of Vital Water

One way to take care of our health would therefore be to drink more EZ-rich water. But how do we get vital, life-enhancing, structured water?

Unless we live near a natural, babbling brook, or a glacier, our water is usually delivered to our homes by a municipal drinking water supply; we can use physical methods to de-cluster our tap water, and thus return it to its original natural state. A simple method for this is swirling with special devices that restructure the water from the pipes in your home. In this process, the cluster formations imposed on the water molecules by standing still or by the water flowing through very long pipes are freed, enriched with energy and oxygen, and rearranged into EZ water that nourishes and invigorates our body cells.

Since my student days, I have been using a drinking water swirler for my drinking water treatment both in our practice clinic and at home. This is connected to the water tap and guides the pressurized water through a special flow form that creates rapidly rotating vortices. A rotation rate of up to 22,700 revolutions per minute has been calculated inside such a drinking water swirler. These rotational forces fling the large-structured, solidified clusters of water apart, thus atomizing or de-clustering it into its original, small-structured and fine cluster structures and thereby charging it with new energy. Water treated in this way maintains its structured state for several hours and can deploy its beneficial effect in our organism when we drink it or when we prepare our food with it. It even tastes better and is easier to drink, as reported by most people to whom I have offered it.

To additionally filter out chemical impurities from the drinking water, one can use an activated carbon filter, for example. Special water shops, which can be found in many larger cities, can advise on this topic. Especially in countries that do not provide safe drinking water or that chlorinate the drinking water, this filtration purification method is highly recommended.

Start each day by drinking a glass (about three hundred milliliters) of fresh and preferably structured, for example, swirled, water. It compensates for the loss of fluids during the night, smooths the skin, improves the flow properties of the blood, stimulates the excretion of toxins, and vitalizes the entire organism. During the day, too, it is important to drink a glass of fresh water every hour, for example, at work, in order to take in the daily required amount of fluid of about 3 liters a day.

3.4 Oxygen, Breathing, and Cancer Growth

> *There are two graces in breathing:*
> *drawing in air, and discharging it.*
> *The former constrains, the latter refreshes:*
> *so marvelously is life mixed.*
> *Thank God then when He presses you,*
> *and thank Him again when He lets you go.*[3]
>
> —JOHANN WOLFGANG VON GOETHE

3.4.1 How Does Cancer Growth Relate to the Oxygen in Our Body?

Our life is inconceivable without breath. Oxygen is needed at every moment of our lives and must be continuously supplied through our breath. At the same time, the combustion product carbon dioxide, which is continuously produced in our mitochondria, must be disposed of through exhalation.

A lack of oxygen (hypoxia) in an organ or tissue of a human being favors the development and the faster, more aggressive growth of cancer cells. These thrive best in the areas with the weakest oxygen supply: in the end-flow areas of the venous capillaries and the tissues adjacent to them. This is the place where the oxygen transported in the blood has already been completely delivered to the tissues and the venous blood is low in oxygen and rich in carbon dioxide. Specifically, it is usually mucosal or glandular tissue cells that then suffer from oxygen deficiency and, after a longer period of time, form a carcinoma (cancerous growth) that is well adapted to the lack of oxygen.

A lack of oxygen in our tissues is in any case one of the essential factors for the aging of the human organism. So aging itself is per se a risk factor for cancer! Due to age-related changes in our blood vessels—deposits and gradual thickening of the vessel walls and their stiffening—as well as inflammatory processes, the diffusion of oxygen from the blood into the tissues is constantly weakening, especially in the end-flow vessels, the capillaries. Stimulating microcirculation and thereby improving the uptake of oxygen into our cells and the mitochondria they contain is therefore an important goal of both antiaging medicine and holistic oncology. Everything that improves the microcirculation in our organism and thus improves the oxygen supply can also help us to prevent cancer, or to make existing cancer cells milder and less aggressive.

In recent years, scientists have described the effects of organ hypoxia in biochemical detail. Oxygen deficiency, hyperacidity, and faster cancer cell growth form a vicious circle. The faster the tumor grows, the more the oxygen deficiency increases. As a result, cancer cells become more and more like sugar-fermenting cells and produce more and more lactic acid (lactate). This leads to tissue overacidification (see section 3.10, "The Acid–Base Balance," page 135) and at the same time to the migration of connective tissue cells into the tumor. The connective tissue cells also change their function in such a way that they serve cancer growth; they become cancer-associated fibroblasts, which can make up as much as 80 percent of a tumor node. Among other things, these altered fibroblasts send out messenger substances that block the immune system in its cancer-fighting function. All this leads, as long as the oxygen deficiency prevails, to a selection of aggressive cancer cells that grow faster and infiltrate the immune system more and more.

Our Breath Keeps Us Healthy

What can we do? How do we breathe in a healthy way? How can we promote our health through breathing exercises and do ourselves additional good through special oxygen therapies?

Let's start with the most natural thing, breathing itself. We can learn to breathe healthily! The modern stressed person usually breathes too shallowly and too quickly. This makes the breath ineffective. The inhaled air does not reach the depth of the lungs where oxygen exchange takes place. The consequences of the resulting lack of oxygen are enormous: from tiredness, to poor concentration, to faster aging and a higher risk of cancer.

Irregular, shallow breathing or—unconsciously—holding one's breath not only leads to oxygen deficiency and its effects on the physical level, but also has consequences on a psychological level: The feeling of anxiety, trepidation, a general malaise, or even an unspecific feeling of compulsion is thus unconsciously increased or evoked.

In certain situations, we may find that something "takes our breath away." This expression indicates the need to gasp, but it is not a helpful way to breathe. In these situations, we are usually lacking steadfastness, verbal clout, and have also run out of good ideas and positive thoughts.

If we breathe shallowly or haltingly for a longer period of time, we may even start to think anxious thoughts that always revolve around the same problems, as if in a spiral, and from which we can't seem to find a way out. In extreme cases, we know this shallow breathing from states of shock, in which the *first aid of breathing*, namely exhaling, is usually appropriate even *before* any medical help is given. After exhaling, inhaling follows as if by itself. Even and regular exhalation and inhalation are usually what is required to counteract panicking.

In her book *Protected, Preserved, Safe* (*Beschützt, bewahrt, geborgen*), Luisa Francia dedicates an entire chapter to exhalation. With a few examples, she describes the importance and consequences of exhaling and is certain: "It is always about the exhale. Because when the breath can flow completely out of the body, you don't have to worry about the inhale anymore." To become free, we should let go of the breath so that we can face the dangers or everyday adversities of life. A controlled exhale, she says, leads to conscious letting go "and the associated escape from mental hamster wheels. The exhale is the overture to freedom, it sheds ballast and gets to the heart of the matter—the inhale."

But in order to use breathing to improve our health and increase our well-being, let's first take a closer look at a few details to understand how we breathe and what happens in the process. The most important breathing muscle is the diaphragm. It is a kind of plate of tendons and muscles and separates the abdominal cavity from the chest cavity, where it is covered by the peritoneum and the pleura respectively. The expansion of the rib cage by the diaphragm and intercostal muscles is controlled involuntarily—we do not have to consciously control our breathing movements—whereupon the lungs are filled with sufficient breathable air.

The two separate lungs have a vascular covering, fill the lateral halves of the chest cavity, and border the pleura.

When we are relaxed and at rest, we breathe in about five hundred milliliters of air through normal diaphragmatic breathing. When we are more active, for example, during exercise, much more air is drawn into the lungs, depending on the oxygen required.

However, in everyday life we may breathe in a very shallow and akinetic manner, without being aware of it. As a result—and also in connection with too little exercise—too little oxygen gets into our bloodstream and into our cells to really be able to promote health. We should therefore expand our normal breathing and practice deeper breathing.

With diaphragmatic breathing, the diaphragm is tensed, lowered, and the lungs are allowed to expand, with air flowing through the lower third of the lungs. The oxygen in the air we breathe is transported from the trachea via the main bronchi into the right and left lungs and from there it is passed on via the bronchi and bronchioles to the alveoli. From there, it diffuses into the blood vessels.

Exhalation follows this muscular process passively and automatically. During this process, the chest cavity and its organs are only slightly stretched or even massaged; the abdominal cavity and its organs remain largely motionless and unstretched.

To stretch the abdominal muscles and move the abdominal organs, we have to breathe with abdominal breathing. Here, the chest cavity enlarges while the abdominal cavity shrinks and the abdominal organs are pushed forward and down. The abdominal wall visibly bulges forward. If we continue to take in air with a long breath after the abdominal wall has already noticeably bulged, flank breathing sets in and the ribs are pulled even further apart and stretched by the diaphragm.

If we replace normal breathing or even pure, shallow chest breathing with deep breathing that moves the abdominal muscles and organs, not only can your voice—and your mood—be improved, digestion is also promoted, the stomach, but above all the intestines, are stimulated, and also the heart, as it sits on the diaphragm, is expanded downwards. As a result, it becomes larger or longer and can absorb more blood from the veins. Together with the subsequent exhalation and the reduction of its original size, the heart is supported in its own muscular cardiac activity. With the help of this conscious abdominal breathing, we can perform an efficient and beneficial organ self-massage on a daily basis. Breathing exercises for relaxation, performed in yoga or gymnastics, are also based on the same principles of movement.

After we have learned to breathe normally again, that is, deeply, with the right muscles and at the right rate and tempo, we can turn to therapies that improve oxygen saturation and more effective microcirculation, the oxygen therapies.

3.4.2 Oxygen Inhalations to Stimulate Microcirculation . . . and Improvement of Oxygen Saturation

The Oxygen Multistep Therapy According to von Ardenne

The oxygen multistep therapy (OMT) was developed by the German physicist Manfred von Ardenne (1907–1997) and applied in Dresden from 1970 onward. Von Ardenne developed it during his collaboration with the Nobel Prize–winner Otto Warburg (1883–1970) and based his own research on his results. By then, the range of his inventions had already extended from radio technology to television and the invention of the scanning electron microscope. From the 1960s onward, von Ardenne became increasingly involved in medical issues and developed new ideas and technologies for the treatment of cancer. He was the first to intensively research and scientifically present the importance of oxygen therapies in oncology, and he was already of the opinion at that time that insufficient oxygen supply to the cells (in old age) was (partly) responsible for the fact that vital processes in the organism no longer run or do not run optimally and that diseases, such as cancer, can develop.

The aim of OMT is to increase the oxygen content of the blood and the organs over a longer period of time and thus favorably influence chronic diseases, improve blood circulation, strengthen the immune system, and increase performance. As the name suggests, the treatment takes place in several steps: First, the patient is administered a vitamin-mineral mixture of vitamin B_1, vitamin C, and magnesium, followed by oxygen inhalation while experiencing an artificially induced fever (hyperthermia). For more information on hyperthermia, see chapter 6.

The Pulsating Electromagnetic Frequency Therapy

Another therapy method to improve the microcirculation and thus the oxygen saturation in tissues is the pulsating electromagnetic frequency therapy, PEMF for short. With the help of oscillating electromagnetic fields, which are transmitted to the human body via a therapy mat or a cushion, microcirculation and oxygen transport are effectively stimulated. This therapy is completely free of side effects and is an important component of holistic cancer medicine. It is also used successfully in the prevention or treatment of many chronic diseases.

After only a few treatments with PEMF, with the help of a dark field microscope one can see how the flow properties of red blood cells change positively (see figures 2 and 3 in the color insert).

The regularly observable resolution of the "rouleaux formation phenomenon" in the dark field microscope after PEMF is explained by the improvement of the electrical membrane potential (normal value at negative ten millivolts) of the blood corpuscles, that is, the electrical charge that every living cell maintains on its surface through the constant transport of charged atoms—ions, such as sodium+ or potassium+. In an organism plagued by oxygen deficiency, smoldering inflammation, or even cancer, the cell membranes of our blood cells also work less effectively, which leads to low cell membrane charge and eventually to sticking of the blood cells, or the rouleaux formation phenomenon. Cells with higher membrane potential repel each other and thus flow better through the vessels without sticking together. This is enormously advantageous for oxygen transport and improves the flow properties of the blood, which has clear advantages, and not only in the case of cancer.

Depending on the severity of the disease, the positive effect visible in the microscope image of a PEMF treatment lasts for hours or even several days. For chronic illnesses, we recommend continuous, or daily, treatment with PEMF.

Oxyvenation Therapy According to Dr. Regelsberger

Another form of therapy that is used in complementary medicine for chronic inflammatory diseases is intravenous oxygen therapy or intravenous oxyvenation therapy (IOT), in which medical oxygen is directly administered into the veins. This procedure was developed in the 1950s by the neurologist/neurosurgeon and oxygen researcher from Detmold, Helmut Regelsberger (1918–1990), and has been carried out in over two hundred thousand individual treatments.

Oxyvenation has a strong anti-inflammatory effect and is based on the principle of *hormesis* (Greek for stimulation, or impetus): Small amounts of pure oxygen are slowly insufflated (pumped) into the arm vein over fifteen to twenty-five minutes via a precision pump. This completely unnatural stimulus exerted by the small oxygen bubbles in the blood stimulates the regulatory capacity of the organism, especially the immune system. Through biochemical reactions in various blood cells that follow the stimulus of the IOT, the blood circulation improves more and more after a few applications. This leads to a number of noticeable and measurable improvements in a variety of diseases.

Positive effects of IOT can be recorded for very different diseases: For example, improvements are seen in circulatory disorders of the heart and voluntary muscles (angina pectoris or intermittent claudication), in allergic diseases, neurodermatitis, bronchial asthma, and also in cancer.

HOW IS THIS POSSIBLE?

The explanation lies in the following biochemical reactions, which have a positive effect in all these different diseases, as the internist and former chairman of the Society for Oxyvenation Therapy, Dr. Frank Kreutzer, summarizes: The body initially treats the small molecular oxygen bubbles like foreign bodies and coats them with a protein film. In this way, they can be absorbed by the eosinophils (special white blood cells that attract the red pigment eosin). This increases the number of these white blood cells, and a modulation of the immune system gradually sets in, which leads to a permanent reduction in inflammation in many chronic inflammatory diseases and allergies.

Furthermore, more prostacyclin (a hormone derived from arachidonic acid) is produced by the tissues, which causes vasodilation and inhibits platelets from sticking together. In addition, the enzymes para oxygenase-1 and haem oxygenase-1 are produced by the organism after IOT stimulation. They have a positive effect on autoimmune diseases. The method has been proven safe and with minimal side effects for seventy years. The only harmless side effect is a slight coughing that lasts for a few minutes after the first treatments. This is due to an overproduction of the tissue hormone bradykinin.

In complementary oncology, IOT is used not least because of its effect of triggering the renewed formation of soluble adhesion molecules. Cancer cells develop properties during their development that support them in their migration (metastasis) through the body. These properties include, among other things, the loss of proteins that sit on the surface of cells and mediate their binding to other cells. Without these adhesion molecules, it is easier for the cancer cells to break free from the surrounding tissue. The renewed formation of the adhesion molecules means that tumor cells are less able to migrate into the tissue and form metastases. IOT therefore has an antimetastatic effect.

3.5 Maintaining Intestinal Health

> *The intestine is the father of all tribulations!*
> *A healthy intestine is the root of all health!*
>
> —HIPPOCRATES

Hippocrates' words emphasize not only the influence of intestinal bacteria on brain chemistry, but also their influence on the entire organism. This claim, which is over two thousand years old, has obviously lost none of its truth, but until the 1990s, both knowledge of and interest in the significance of the microorganisms (bacteria, viruses, fungi, and parasites) living in our organism, the microbiome, was minimal.

In the last three decades, however, the growing scientific interest in and the research published on our microbiome have provided entirely new and impressive insights that are of great importance for our health and the prevention and treatment of diseases. The intestine, with its significance for the physical and the psychological, therefore occupies an important place in the overall structure of the vital field theory.

If we look at the history of man and his microbiome, we see that we have changed it just as drastically as our social life in the last one hundred to two hundred years through changes in lifestyle and diet. For a long time, from the primitive forms of man to the beginning of the industrial age, we humans were surrounded by *dirt* and the microbes it contained. There were no antibacterial soaps, no running water or antibiotics, and we ingested food that was anything but sterile. Today, most people suffer the consequences of sterility, of a bacteria-free diet and excessive hygiene. The result is an insufficient colonization of the intestine by vital symbionts, beneficial microorganisms that help us to stay healthy and without which we would not even be able to live. Some of our intestinal bacteria, if we still have them, regulate inflammatory processes as well as the immunological defense against cancer and even parts of tumor cell spread. They also influence our food metabolism and have an impact on the stability of our genes. The importance of our microbiome for our health is probably as great as that of our genome (the totality of our genetic makeup), and the quality and diversity of our intestinal flora (intestinal microbiome) correlates significantly to our life expectancy.

3.5.1 Balance and Specialization

Certain body regions, such as the gastrointestinal tract, the skin, the nasal cavity, the vagina, hair follicles, the prostate, the mammary glands, and others, have their own specific microbiome. Many of the microorganisms within them are commensals (from the Latin for *sitting at the same table*) that live in us but do not provide us with any particular advantage. Symbiotic bacteria are those with which we have a mutual cooperation. They benefit from us by us providing them with the entire living environment, such as intestinal surface, pH value of the surroundings, food, and so forth. In return, the bacteria ferment our digested food.

The bacterial balance is crucial for health and disease and is one of the most important prerequisites of homeostasis, not only of our immune system but also of our entire organism. What is healthy in balance or in one region, can trigger a disease in another region or when there is too much. Too little of certain microorganisms is not ideal either.

For example, there are bacteria that are harmless in the nasal cavity, but can cause a serious infection in the lungs. If, for example, tissue is injured or the intestinal flora is disturbed by antibiotics, certain microorganisms can become pathogenic. The stomach bacterium *Helicobacter pylori* can also cause inflammation of the stomach's mucous membrane (gastritis) in certain circumstances. This can even lead significantly to the development of stomach cancer, but interestingly, a certain amount of these bacteria protects against reflux disease and esophageal cancer. Here, too, it becomes clear that the right balance is the key to health.

3.5.2 The Microbiome

The term *microbiome* refers to the sum of all microorganisms (such as bacteria and other unicellular organisms) that are resident in a particular habitat, in this case on or in the human body. These are more foreign cells than human ones: An inconceivably large proportion, in fact 90 percent, of the cells that make up our bodies are made up of these nonhuman microorganisms such as bacteria, viruses, protozoa, fungi, and archaea. In fact, we are made up of ten times more microorganisms than human body cells! The weight of our microbiome is roughly comparable to that of our brain, 1.5 kilograms.

The composition of our microbiome is formed primarily in the first three years of life. In the womb, the baby and its intestine are still sterile (germ-free). Only during natural, vaginal birth does the infant come into contact with the bacterial colonization in the birth canal with billions of bacteria from the mother, which cover the infant's body everywhere. This infant also receives their first "oral vaccination" through the mother's vaginal secretions and comes into contact with the germs of the rest of the environment directly after birth.

Children who are born by caesarean section are at a disadvantage due to the absence of bacteria foreign to the organism, and they may later have a higher risk of disease due to a weaker immune system.

For this reason, especially in the United States, Australia, and Great Britain, subsequent vaccination with the mother's vaginal secretion is practiced by rubbing it into the newborn in order to strengthen their immune system. The effect and the positive impact of the *vaginal seeding* has not, however, been researched in long-term studies and is viewed with skepticism in many countries.

There is no doubt that medical progress and the minimization of health risks for mother and child through caesarean delivery are extremely positive. But if a caesarean section is only performed because this form of childbirth is already common practice in some countries and social classes, or because it is easy to plan, for example, for scheduling reasons, the mother may be depriving the child of a significant experience.

Our microbiome is the most important "training camp" for our immune system, and the intestinal microbes are its most important trainers. Up to 80 percent of our immune cells are located in the intestine, especially in the mucous membranes of the small and large intestine. Without our microbiome, our immune system cannot mature at all and make the complicated selection decisions about what to attack and what not to attack. Immunological confusion occurs when the microbiome does not provide the appropriate terrain for our immune system: Allergies, infections, and autoimmune diseases can be the result.

The microbiome is also involved in detoxification processes, with regard to both foreign substances and the organism's own hormones. In addition to digestion, it is also significantly involved in the absorption, synthesis, and activation of vitamins—such as vitamin B_{12}, vitamin K, and folic acid, which are produced by lactic acid bacteria.

While we have about a hundred different intestinal bacteria in infancy, the number of microorganisms living in our intestines reaches about a thousand in adulthood. In old age, the bacterial variability decreases again, which is associated with aging processes and dwindling vitality.

Antibiotic treatments, chronic stress, chemotherapy, and especially an unhealthy diet, including not enough symbiotic bacteria and dietary fibers (see also section 3.2, "Healthy Nutrition and Health-Promoting Dietary Supplements Using the Example of the Twelve Vital Fields," page 36) also have a damaging effect on our microbiome.

3.5.3 The Gut–Brain Axis

It has been known for only a few years that the gut and especially its microbiome interacts intimately with the brain. The gut does indeed "think." And we should also pay attention to this by listening to our *gut feeling*. Our gut bacteria also influence mental health; Hippocrates' idea has been confirmed by numerous researchers. So far, a number of correlations have been established between specific gut bacteria, their metabolites, and neurological symptoms. But how exactly the intestinal flora influences our behavior, our memory, and also diseases such as anxiety disorders or depression, is the subject of ongoing research.

The research has previously shown that altering the composition of the gut microbiota can change neurobiochemistry and that, for example, certain bacteria were found to be reduced in people with depression. A Belgian study published in the magazine *Nature* in 2019 described how the intestinal flora of 1,063 subjects was examined for such bacteria that interact with the central nervous system. The scientists found two groups of bacteria—*Coprococcus* and *Dailister*—that were lowered in people suffering from depression. This showed a positive correlation between the study factor "quality of life" and the ability of the microbiome to synthesize a specific substance that is a breakdown product of the neurotransmitter dopamine. When it was published in 2019, this study was considered the strongest evidence that our microbiome is involved in our emotions and neurological processes.

However, the interactions discovered so far between the gut and the brain work both ways. For example, it has been proven that the microbiome can either produce or modulate the production of the neurotransmitters serotonin, GABA (gamma-aminobutyric acid), and dopamine. These neurotransmitters can also alter the growth of intestinal bacteria. It is a complex world that is created by the interaction of the trillions of gut bacteria with our body cells. The clear functional boundary between the gut and the brain is becoming increasingly blurred in these areas.

3.5.4 **Intestinal Flora, Blood Sugar, and the Microbiome in Cancer**

In 2019, the renowned scientific journal *PNAS* published a study from Columbia University in New York. It described the involvement of the intestinal microbiome in the regulation of blood sugar through the production of the messenger substance serotonin. This finding is just as important for the widespread disease diabetes mellitus (diabetes in adults) as it is for obesity. Both diseases significantly increase the risk of developing cancer. For years now, there has even been talk of a cancer-specific oncobiome, as was described for ovarian cancer in a publication from 2017. Ovarian cancer tumors show a typical constellation of virus parasites and bacterial contamination. Future studies will hopefully be able to show in more detail how this organ-specific oncobiome is related to the gut microbiome. It is already clear today that good gut health or taking a probiotic has a positive effect on oncological treatments. A placebo-controlled study at the University Hospital in Vienna showed that positive modulation of the microbiome through oral administration of a probiotic—consisting of four *Lactobacillus* strains during chemotherapy of breast cancer patients—led to a significant improvement in the quality of life and a reduction in the side effects of vaginal syndrome (vaginitis with dryness, fungal infection, and functional impairment). The positive influence of a multispecies probiotic with ten different intestinal symbionts on the response to chemotherapy in ovarian cancer patients was also documented at the Charité University Hospital in Berlin. The probiotic was administered parallel to chemotherapy. Similar studies in lymphoma patients receiving chemotherapy came to the same conclusion.

We recommend that all patients take a probiotic parallel to chemotherapy, preferably after prior examination of the intestinal microbiome by means of a stool sample, in order to selectively give the symbiotic bacteria that are important for the particular patient at the time.

3.5.5 **When the Gut Leaks: Leaky Gut Syndrome**

The upper part of our digestive system was called the *hypochondrium* in ancient medicine, which refers to the region of the lower ribs. From this, however, the term *hypochondriac* underwent a change of meaning and was eventually used in modern medicine to refer to people who were often resistant to ordinary treatments and had a fear of suffering from a (more) serious illness without being able to find its cause.

For a few years now, the *hypochondrium*, or the upper digestive tract, has increasingly become the focus of modern medicine and is once again experiencing a change in meaning: The digestive tract is—more often than we think—the cause or at least one of the causes of many common diseases. The term *leaky gut* has attracted a lot of attention recently and is currently the subject of intensive research.

Our digestive tract provides an internal surface area of approximately four hundred square meters with which we can absorb nutrients. Leaky gut syndrome occurs when the connections between the intestinal mucosa cells open due to bacterial miscolonization in the intestine and/or chronic inflammation of the intestinal mucosa, resulting in wounds, holes, or tears. Through them, substances from the intestine can get into the blood that should not be there (in this molecular size). Normally, our intestinal mucosal barrier allows only very small molecules to pass through and directs them from the intestine into the lymphatic and blood vessels. Larger substances/molecules instead remain in the intestine to be either excreted or further digested.

However, if molecules have exceeded a certain size and entered the bloodstream due to the permeability of the intestinal mucosal barrier, they trigger an inflammatory reaction in the organism. A leaky gut is often the result of the typical Western diet with too little fiber, too much sugar, and saturated fatty acids. Stress, certain medications, and excessive alcohol consumption also promote the formation of the leaky gut. Tragically, the consequences of a leaky gut fuel further inflammatory reactions, which in turn can lead to food intolerances (IgG4 hypersensitivity reactions). These intolerances in turn trigger or can exacerbate autoimmune diseases. A true vicious circle of more and more unwanted and senseless inflammation that keeps coming back.

Some studies already indicate a link between autoimmune diseases, such as lupus (tissue rheumatism), type 1 diabetes, multiple sclerosis, chronic fatigue syndrome, fibromyalgia, arthritis, asthma, acne, obesity, and neurological diseases. Further studies and research are needed to better understand these relationships.

This lapse can be measured by determining a carbohydrate in the stool, zonulin. If zonulin levels are found to be too high in a stool sample, this indicates a leaky gut syndrome, and measures can be taken to cure it.

Figurately speaking, leaky gut syndrome could also be seen as a weak link between me (what belongs in my blood and what doesn't) and the environment (what is already in my gut but still needs to be digested to become *mine*). No distinction and appropriate reaction to it is possible; altogether too much and too little of the adapted *environment* is absorbed into my blood, which triggers a defense reaction. But this in turn can become a disease, because it does not remedy the weakness of my filter, in this case the intestinal barrier.

How to counteract the leaky gut and reverse the spiral of the disease can be found in chapter 6.

3.6 Stress

The World Health Organization names stress as the greatest health threat of the twenty-first century and "the leading cause of premature death in Europe," as quoted by the Swedish heart specialist and stress researcher Peter Währborg in his book *Stress och den nya ohälsan* (*Stress and the New Unhealthiness*). Stress is directly associated with cardiovascular disease, respiratory disease, impaired sexual function, and all complex diseases such as cancer. Many people today feel stressed for long periods of time in their lives. One occupational group that particularly suffers from stress at work is young cancer specialists, the oncologists. According to recent studies, the rate of oncologists who suffer from burnout syndrome as a result of chronic stress is as high as 70 percent.

3.6.1 What Stress Is and Where It Can Come From

The word *stress* is of English origin and means "tension, pressure, burden." The term was introduced into medicine by the Hungarian-Canadian physician and hormone researcher Hans Selye (1907–1982). In 1,700 papers and a total of thirty-nine books, he dealt with the phenomenon of stress, founded a stress research institute, and ensured that most of the world's languages have adopted the word *stress*.

For Selye, stress is the adaptation reaction of humans to certain stimuli, called stressors, through their perception and interpretation. Stress researchers, neurologists, and immunologists following Selye have outlined further connections between the central stress organ, the brain, and the endocrine glands that communicate with the immune system.

The hypothalamic-pituitary-adrenal axis (HPA axis, also called *stress axis*) leads to a change in the basic function of the entire organism after permanent activation by stressors (see figure 3.2). After a certain period of permanent stress, the brain assumes that a stressful situation will last longer and that overload represents the normal state, even before this has become true. This principle is called *allostasis*, which translates as "achieving stability through change." Here, possible future stresses are incorporated into physiological and psychological behavior to ensure stability even if the stress continues. Complex problems and the anticipation of future stresses by our brain change the basis of our emergency responses. The former *emergency mode* with increased muscle tone, shallower and faster breathing, and increased irritability, among other things, becomes the new "normal state."

––––––––––

If the actual demand for energy exceeds the supply of the organism over a longer period of time (stress), the brain, its appendage gland (pituitary gland), and the subordinate adrenal glands adapt and secrete more stress hormones such as adrenaline, noradrenaline, testosterone, and cortisol. Gradually, an *allostatic* load builds up that is tantamount to an overload. It leads to faster wear and tear of the entire organism with increased risk for most of our modern civilization diseases: heart attacks, vascular diseases, sleep disorders, depression, and cancer. These diseases occur more frequently when the allostatic load has been too great for a long time.

In this day and age, social factors play the most important role in this drama: The strongest or most effective stressors are belittlement, indignity, discrimination, and stigmatization, those situations that are associated with feelings of shame and humiliation. A clear correlation between social and health situations is noted worldwide. Health inequalities, including different chances of recovery or of staying healthy, have their roots here. The prevalence of severe stress decreases with increasing socioeconomic status: It falls from 17.3 percent with low socioeconomic status to 7.6 percent with high socioeconomic status. If there is little social support, it even rises to 26 percent. Women report a high stress level significantly more often (13.9 percent) than men do (8.2 percent).

One scientific field of research focuses on this interaction of stress and disease: Psychoneuroimmunology (PNI) or psychoimmunology is an interdisciplinary field of science that deals with the interaction of the psyche,

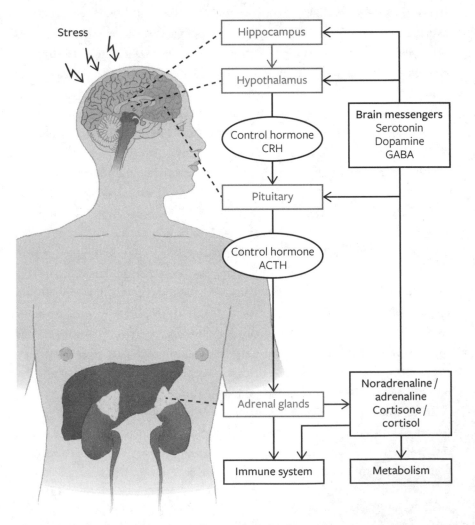

Figure 3.2. The hypothalamic-pituitary-adrenal axis.

the nervous system, and the immune system. In psychoneuroendocrinology (PNE), the hormone system is also included, and in psycho-oncology, the significance for cancer diseases.

An important discovery that led to the emergence of PNI as a new scientific discipline was the realization that messenger substances of the nervous system have an effect on the immune system and, conversely, that messenger substances of the immune system have an effect on the nervous system. The influence therefore takes place from both sides.

Certain messenger substances, the neuropeptides from the pituitary gland, can dock onto immune cells (for example, macrophages) and influence them in terms of both speed and direction of movement. Put simply, this means that our brain activity influences the control and function of our immune cells (see also section 3.4, "Oxygen, Breathing, and Cancer Growth," page 82).

It has also been clearly shown how chronic stress lowers the concentration of immune substances (immunoglobulin A) in saliva, and this leads to increased release of adrenal hormones (glucocorticoids) that inhibit the immune system (for example, cytokine production, and reactivity of T and B lymphocytes and natural killer cells). The tendency to suppress anger instead of expressing it, and higher levels of anxiety and depression, lead to measurable negative changes in our immune system. Acute stress can increase the performance of the nonspecific, innate immune system within minutes. Chronic stress does the opposite! It lowers the performance of both the innate and the adaptive immune systems through general immunosuppression or leads to immune dysfunction, such as silent inflammation (see section 3.12, "Chronic Inflammation: Silent Inflammation," page 150). All this contributes to a higher risk of developing cancer.

Stress from gainful employment and particularly high pressure in terms of social status and lifestyle are very pronounced in some cultures. In Japan, for example, there is a special word for "death from overworking": *karoshi*. In 2013, the death of a thirty-one-year-old journalist made headlines because she was found dead in bed after working 159 hours of overtime in one month. She was not suffering from any known illness. Her organism collapsed due to overworking.

What we perceive as a stressor and what we don't is also influenced by the programming or imprinting of our brain during the first six to eight years of life. During this period of our childhood, our brain is in a kind of *cognitive trance*, storing everything that is offered to it. Deep-seated behavioral patterns, including, for example, feelings of guilt or shame, usually have their origin in childhood experiences and imprints that accompany our perception of ourselves, the world, and stress throughout our lives. As long as we do not recognize this, these behavioral patterns continue to influence us as adults. However, we can change our behavior and how we deal with it through self-education or therapy.

A very successful form of therapy that can positively change programming from childhood is hypnotherapy. It was introduced into clinical psychiatry between the 1950s and 1980s by the American psychiatrist Milton Erickson (1901–1980) and is now practiced by hypnotherapists all over the world.

3.6.2 Coping with Cancer

How people deal with and cope with cancer is called a *coping strategy*. This is something which can be learned, as well as improved. However, psycho-oncology also deals with the context of how a person with cancer can influence the progression of the disease by changing their inner attitude and outer lifestyle. In her groundbreaking book *Radical Remission: Surviving Cancer Against All Odds*, the American medical scientist Kelly Turner, PhD, impressively demonstrated that seven out of nine factors influencing cancer are of a psychoemotional or spiritual nature. Turner gathered this from over a thousand interviews with advanced cancer patients who, contrary to the assumption of the treating oncologists, were able to achieve a sustained remission (decline of the disease) through their inner attitude and the way they dealt with cancer.

The remaining two of the nine factors listed consisted of dietary changes and the intake of natural substances. In chapter 6, Kelly Turner's nine factors are explained as examples of practice and imitation.

Whether we perceive something as a stressor or not is—as mentioned above—related to our experiences, our individual perception, and their interpretation. Obviously, however, this framework has changed decisively in the past one hundred years. Stress in this impacting form seems to be a problem of the modern era and modern industrial nations. Compared to everything that humanity has gone through before in terms of change, what we humans have gone through in the recent past and how we see and behave in relation to our environment has changed our relationship to the world around us. Above all, the speed at which we have changed or even destroyed our own environment (nature) in the last one hundred to two hundred years through industrial invention ultimately confronts us with the questions of how and with what aspiration we can cope with the pressures we impose on ourselves.

We perceive ourselves and the world around us in a way that has never occurred before in all the millennia of human cultural history. Never before have we processed and "done" so much in such a short time. The speed at which we live and fulfill our tasks has increased enormously in the last one hundred years.

The sociologist and Jena University professor Hartmut Rosa presented the problem in detail in his 2004 postdoctoral thesis on social acceleration. Alongside automation and mechanization, fast food, speed dating, multitasking, and power napping are phenomena of an era when there is not enough time and everything has to be done quickly and effectively. Terms such as *enhancement compulsion* and *shrinking of the present* are characteristic of our everyday life. At the same time, the ever-increasing number of sensory impressions that our brain has to process every day leads to a complete sensory overload and an increase in the allostatic load described above. The omnipresent smartphone with its multitude of signals, which constantly draws our attention to it, and the social media on which we document our lives and post and "like" a seemingly limitless number of seemingly important but actually often very banal updates, are increasingly draining our lifetime and vital energy. In the process, our real encounters are impoverished and time with ourselves is increasingly lost.

The countermovement to this can be found, for example, in books like *Now*, by Eckhart Tolle. We are called to find ourselves and the *now* in which life actually takes place. In a modern way and without using the concept of God, Tolle demonstrates what could already be found two thousand years before him in the wisdom teachings of the great world religions. This is also one of the central messages of the Chinese philosopher Lao Tse (probably sixth century BC), who, as the founder of Taoism, taught this thousands of years ago in the work attributed to him, *Tao Te Ching*:

> *When everyone knows beauty as beauty,*
> *Ugliness arises,*
> *When everyone knows good as good,*
> *Evil arises,*
> *Thus:*
> *Being and non-being produce each other,*
> *Difficult and easy complement each other,*
> *Long and short define each other,*
> *High and low support each other,*
> *Music and voice harmonise with each other,*
> *Before and after follow each other.*
> *Therefore, the wise man acts without deeds,*
> *Teaches without words,*
> *Things flourish without resistance,*
> *He lets them prosper and does not possess them,*
> *He does nothing and demands nothing for himself,*
> *And does not take anything for himself, from what he accomplishes,*
> *And because he does not take anything,*
> *He does not lose anything.*
>
> —Lao Tse, *Tao Te Ching*[4]

You have to study these 2,600-year-old words for a while to decipher their deeper meaning. They seem strange to us today in the prevailing pressures of being oriented toward performance, goal fulfillment, and effectiveness, but they reveal their deeper meaning or truth in prolonged occupation with them or in meditation on them.

The founders of Zen Buddhism in the fifth century AD, influenced by Lao Tse, as well as the tradition of Jesus in the Sermon on the Mount, also point us to an essential aspect of life: live in trust in what is, now, in the present. "Therefore do not worry about tomorrow, for tomorrow will take care of itself."[5]

The experience of being and of being completely absorbed in the present is a source of strength of a fundamental kind that we can still observe in children every day, but that has been lost to most adults and to modern man in general. We can, however, find our way back to the now, to the experience of being, by becoming aware of ourselves again and by living in the moment again and again, ideally for once without words and deeds, without resistance and wanting, without doing and having to do.

In his book *Resonance: A Sociology of Modernity* (*Resonanz—eine Soziologie der Moderne*), Hartmut Rosa looked at the change that modern man has experienced in his relationship to the world and he came to this conclusion: Modern man is no longer in resonance with the world. The coherence of our lives is increasingly faltering, leading to a discoherence plagued by chronic stress. Rosa defined three fields as axes of resonance in which we relate to the world: the horizontal resonance axis, consisting of family, friendship, and politics; the diagonal axis of resonance, consisting of relationships to the objects around us—our consumer behavior and especially sport and entertainment are attempts to feel ourselves in a world that is becoming more and more abstract—and the vertical axis of resonance, consisting of religion, nature, art, and history. On all levels of the relationship to the world, he stated in eight hundred pages, modern man's ability to oscillate has diminished, and compensatory mechanisms are at work. Is cancer a biological consequence of this?

3.6.3 Mindfulness against Stress

Practicing mindfulness is the most effective way to reduce stress, and I recommend it regularly to my patients. Mindfulness meditation was significantly researched in the West by the American stress researcher and molecular biologist Jon Kabat-Zinn and integrated into the therapy offered by Western stress management programs. Kabat-Zinn founded the Stress Reduction Clinic at the University of Massachusetts in 1979. Empirical knowledge from the study of Zen Buddhism and yoga were integrated into scientific findings about our molecular biological stress reactions. Mindfulness-based stress reduction, MBSR for short, is now practiced and taught in clinics and health institutions around the world. Chapter 6 presents the most important elements of MBSR.

One of the Zen stories that I find the most beautiful, which highlights the principle of nonjudgment—one of the core themes of mindfulness practice—is the following:

The Zen Master Hakuin was praised by his neighbors as someone who lived a pure life. A beautiful Japanese girl whose parents owned a grocery shop lived near him. One day, the parents discovered that their daughter was pregnant. This made them very angry. She did not want to confess who the father was. But after much insistence, she finally named Hakuin. The furious parents confronted the master. "Is that so?" was all he had to say.

After the child was born, they took it to Hakuin. He had lost his reputation, but this did not worry him, and he took care of the child in the best possible way. He received milk and everything else the baby needed from his neighbors.

A year later, the young mother could stand it no longer. She told her parents the truth, that the real father was a young man who worked at the fish market. The girl's mother and father went back to Hakuin and asked for his forgiveness. They apologized profusely and wanted to take the child back. Hakuin agreed. While handing over the child, all he said was "Is that so?"

What this story illustrates in a very subtle and sensitive way is that, according to the current state of science, 95 percent of all chronic diseases are related to stress or are caused or even triggered by stress.

Stress researchers report that 95 percent of the factors that trigger stress are based on our attitude, our interpretation of the situation. Only 5 percent of these factors are based solely on external facts. Stress therefore arises in our own consciousness, through the evaluation of sensations and the feeling: "I can't do it anymore . . . I have to do more, even faster, immediately . . . everything . . . always . . . the same . . . I am responsible . . . If I don't do it now . . . It's all my fault . . ." and so on. The point of origin of stress is the brain, which acts on hormones and the immune system. The longer people are in a state of stress, the weaker their ability to compensate for stress becomes. A control loop with negative feedback is created, what is commonly called a *vicious circle*. In the long term, stress thus leads to a change in the psychoneuroendocrine system and the immune system.

————

One of the most striking examples of what stress can do to our consciousness and our organism is a 1936 case report by N. S. Yawger titled "Emotions as the Cause of Rapid and Sudden Death." In this paper, Yawger cited the case of a young man sentenced to death who—without knowing it—was subjected to a psychological experiment. The man sentenced to death for murder was told that he would avoid the ignominious execution by public hanging and that the death penalty would be carried out by bleeding to death. So he was led into a silent room where, after a blindfold was put on, he now believed the veins in his wrist were to be opened with a sharp instrument. What he did not know was that the instrument was blunt and not a single drop of blood escaped from him. But at the same moment that the supposed cut was made, a vessel filled with water was opened to make a continuous dripping sound, causing the condemned man to hypnotically believe that he was bleeding to death. The report ends with the words: "Although of a strong constitution, the condemned man fainted and then died without losing a drop of blood."

————

This story shows so convincingly how strongly imagination under hypnosis can affect bodily functions that the Swiss psychotherapist and psychologist Gary Bruno Schmid quotes it as an introduction to his textbook on hypnotherapy, *Self-Healing by Imagination*.[6] If this is possible, then we can also assume a health-damaging effect of a carelessly communicated prognosis, which acts on those affected like a prophecy of approaching and certain death. And if the effect of our imagination and beliefs is so powerful, real, and immense, then we should use it to consciously strengthen our health and integrate this into all methods of therapy.

In chapter 6, you will find practical advice on how to work with affirmations and visualizations and strengthen your health.

The Kiel University (in Germany) professor, psychotherapist, and physician Thomas Küchler published one of the most spectacular studies on the topic of "Effects of Psycho-Oncological Measures on the Survival Time of Cancer Patients." It was conducted between 1991 and 1993 at the University Clinic in Hamburg, Germany, and the results were published for the first time in 1999. In 2007, it was published again after another examination of the long-term effect of the treatments, and together with the results of the ten-year survival time of the patients.

In this clinical study, 271 patients suffering from cancer of the digestive organs, all of whom were treated with standard oncology therapies, were randomly divided into two groups. One group received psychotherapeutic care in the form of supportive talks, psychotherapeutic crisis interventions, and introduction to relaxation techniques on an average of twenty-two days in addition to and parallel to the standard therapies in the hospital.

The focus was on passing on information (psychoeducational interventions). Bringing life into balance, expressing existential questions such as fears for the future and expectations, as well as perceiving and expressing feelings were the main topics of this group. Dealing with death and nonverbal communication were also addressed. The aim of the study was to find out whether psychotherapeutic support would positively change and be measurable in the quality of life of the subjects in the treated group (compared to the control group, which received only standard oncological therapies).

Surprisingly, it turned out that a significant difference in survival figures was already evident two years after completion of the psychotherapeutic support. Of the patients who did not receive psycho-oncological support, 33.3 percent (45 patients) were still alive after two years, compared to 50.7 percent (69 patients) of those who received psycho-oncological support. After ten years, the participants in both groups were examined again. In the psycho-oncology group, 21.3 percent (29 patients) were still alive, while of the control group, 9.6 percent (13 patients) were still alive. How is it possible that psycho-oncological support with an average of four hours of therapist contact (222 minutes according to the study) more than doubles the ten-year survival rate of cancer patients?

Since the study was published in the renowned *Journal of Clinical Oncology* and was conducted at the university hospitals in Kiel and Hamburg, we can assume that it was conducted and documented correctly. And since the patients were randomly assigned to the two groups, the findings of the study have a particularly high significance. In brief: Psycho-oncological measures with an average of four hours per patient have the potential to more than double survival time within ten years. The psychobiological causes that lead to this are the subject of PNI.

The original goal of the study, to inspire more hope, find goals, express feelings, and fuel the will to survive through this support, and thus improve the quality of life, was obviously achieved. It resulted in more than doubling the survival rate. However, this also implies that the change in the consciousness of the study participants had a direct effect on the physical, immunological, and tumor-specific factors. The change in the patients' thoughts, feelings, and actions led to the brain and its subordinate endocrine glands and the immune system regulating the signaling substances, immune modulators, and hormone secretion in such a way that physically measurable changes took place that either caused the cancer cells to die or at least effectively increased the organism's ability to control them, up to more than 120 percent prolonged overall survival of the treatment group after ten years.

In comparison, the measurable effect of chemotherapy on the five-year survival of patients with metastatic breast, colorectal, prostate, or lung cancer is, according to an Australian study from 2004, 2.3 to 2.5 percent.

3.6.4 Change Needs Goals

For everyday life, it is important for all of us to clearly sort out, understand, and distribute the responsibilities for the individual areas of life. Helpful questions for this are: What am I solely responsible for? What am I jointly responsible for (together with others)? What am I not responsible for at all?

I advise my patients to write down a list of responsibilities and then sort them into these three categories. Discovering that there is a category three, not being responsible, is often a beneficial insight that should be practiced and deepened!

Even though the term is almost a tongue twister, there is a deep truth in it: *incompetence-compensation-competence*. According to Odo Marquard (philosopher and professor from Gießen, Germany), this should be practiced in order to eliminate the "growing meaning and resistance of the leftovers" and to see the world again with the right interpretation and the right proportions of meaning. Acting according to this is essential for modern man in order not to be constantly drowned in the stress of stimulus overload and the trap of exaggerating nonperfect aspects of our lives. In the vernacular, it is also called "letting things slide."

———

Oscar Carl Simonton, MD, pioneer of psycho-oncology and American radio-oncologist, was one of the first doctors who wrote books since the 1970s on lifestyle changes, health-oriented life planning, a healthy attitude toward life and death, inner work with visualization, hypnosis, and meditation. He held seminars for cancer patients all over the world. I owe my introduction to systematic, psycho-oncological work to him, which I have been incorporating into my work since training in his seminars in 2000.

3.7 Sugar: Cancer Driver of the First Order

The experience of sweetness is something very special. It evokes a multitude of pleasant feelings in us. Satisfaction, strength, and even a certain sense of being with ourselves. A bit of dextrose often helps with physical weakness, and a few pieces of chocolate, preferably with a high cocoa content of at least 80 percent, help with a mild depressive mood.

In Indian tantra philosophy, the word *dhisthana* is translated as both "at home" and "sweetness." The second chakra, or energy center, is called "Swa-Dhisthana" there: *Swa* in Sanskrit means "one's own." *Swa-Dhisthana* is the "sweet own/the home," with its seat in the sacral area, which gives this body region of the deep pelvis another sacred note (*sacrum* comes from Latin and stands for *sanctuary* and *sacrifice*). Is this why we long for so many sweet experiences, which we satisfy with more and more sugar, because we no longer perceive our *home* and our *being with ourselves* as sweet, as pleasant and present?

For thousands of years, sugar was a rare treat for humans, expensive and available only in very small quantities, usually extracted from fruits. A special form of sweetness has been consumed for millennia as honey, which to this day is probably one of the healthiest forms of sweet enjoyment, as it is much more than just sugar or sugary sweet. Enjoyed in moderation, honey is a healthy food and even a remedy.

Honey also consists largely of sucrose. This form of sugar is a carbohydrate that is made up of two sugar molecules (disaccharide). Colloquially, this form of sugar is also called table sugar, crystal sugar, or simply sugar. This type of sugar is mainly obtained from sugar beet, sugar cane, or the sugar palm. The phloem sap contained in sucrose also forms the basis of honey, which the honeybee collects either directly from the nectar of plants or indirectly as honeydew from phloem-sucking insects, such as aphids or cicadas, and transforms into honey by means of a special metabolism in its stomach.

Until the beginning of the industrial age in the nineteenth century, pure sugar was hardly accessible to the general population. Today, people in Germany consume about 40 kilograms per person per year. That is just under 125 grams of granulated sugar per day! This amount is estimated to be twenty times higher than 150 years ago. As early as 2009, the American Heart Association recommended reducing daily consumption to 30 grams for women and 45 grams for men in order to reduce the risk of cardiovascular diseases (stroke and heart attack were the main cause of death). In the United States in particular, per capita consumption of sugar is one of the highest in the world: The average American eats 68 kilograms of white sugar per year.

The most dangerous sources of sugar are all lemonades, ice teas, and cola drinks, which contain around ten grams of sugar per one hundred milliliter of drink. That is one hundred grams of sugar per liter, and such a drink thus contains an average of thirty-five lumps of sugar per liter! It doesn't help when manufacturers—driven by a campaign a few years ago—reduce the amount of sugar in soft drinks by 10 percent. The manufacturers of Coca-Cola made "huge efforts" in 2017 and announced an amended and "reduced-sugar" recipe, which contains "only" thirty-one sugar cubes per liter—which makes no difference to the effect and is still far too much sugar!

Sugar is a drug. Indeed. It not only affects the body, but also our consciousness, our psyche. Sugar can be addictive, and when we stop eating it or greatly reduce our consumption, it can produce withdrawal symptoms that make a relapse into addictive consumption a serious problem. Worldwide, the sugar problem is of greater health significance than all other drugs combined. Yet the sugar drug is easy to get everywhere, cheaply and legally. Even children consume this drug to an almost unlimited extent.

It is now considered undisputed that excessive sugar consumption worldwide directly or indirectly promotes the following diseases: obesity, cardiovascular diseases (such as high blood pressure, heart attacks, or strokes), vascular diseases, type 2 diabetes, depression, caries, fatty liver, gout, arthritis, and, finally, also cancer. High sugar consumption is also responsible for hyperactive behavior (not only in children), premature aging of the skin, acne, chronic fatigue syndrome, and kidney problems.

Sugar (glucose) is absorbed up to fifty times faster by cancer cells than by healthy cells. It has long been regarded as their favorite food and thus promotes their growth and spread. This is why a special form of sugar is also used to diagnose cancer: For examination by the PET (positron emission tomography), patients are injected with sugar together with a weak radioactive substance in order to mark cancer cells. The fluorodeoxyglucose, which is radioactive for only a short time, is absorbed by the cancer cells within a few minutes and accumulates in them much more than in healthy cells. The biochemical functions in the body can thus be made visible by the radioactive radiation as yellow-orange colored regions. In PET-CT, positron emission tomography and computer tomography (CT) are combined in a single device in order to be able to localize and assess healthy and diseased tissue (marked in color by PET) very clearly through the very precise imaging of CT.

The unit of measurement for the radiologist in this assessment of the PET-CT is the SUV (standardized uptake value), which describes the glucose metabolism of a tumor—or more generally, the glucose uptake value of a tissue. If this uptake value is increased, a disease is present. Incidentally, this increased uptake of the radioactive sugar also applies to inflamed cells, which is why it is difficult and sometimes impossible to distinguish between inflammation and cancer in PET-CT, which in turn illustrates the proximity of inflammation and cancer. Therefore, a healthy—meaning moderate—sugar consumption is extremely important for a healthy life!

Sugar can be replaced in its *stimulating function* in many ways, for example, by fresh fruit or dried fruit, and these contribute to health both purely as a snack or dessert and in muesli, yogurt, and quark dishes, main courses, and much more.

However, it can (and unfortunately must) also be clearly stated that it is only healthy if sugar (in its entirety) is consumed in moderation. Nevertheless, another question arises for many of us.

3.7.1 Are Sugar Substitutes the Way Out?

There are a large number of sugar substitutes on the market worldwide, some of which can be more dangerous than sugar itself. They are divided into sweeteners and sugar alcohols. What they all have in common is that they have no or negligible nutritional value, that is, hardly any kilocalories per gram. This makes them seemingly attractive to those who want to reduce carbohydrates in their diet or want to lose weight. They are therefore advertised in countless "diet products." But are they a better choice than sugar?

Sweeteners are found in the vast majority of "light" or diet products, which our organism excretes either completely or largely unchanged. In themselves, they cause a small increase of blood sugar and insulin levels in the blood. Their main disadvantage is, however, that our body does not know what to do with them. The consequence is that the organism does not detoxify them in the best possible way, and these substances do not satisfy the craving for sweet things. The desire for (even more) sweetness remains. The American professor of medicine Helen Hazuda was able to show through her research that people who drank Diet Coke and the like gained 70 percent more weight than those who drank normal sugary soft drinks. The fact that sweeteners are fattening is no longer a secret. The American Heart Association says: "You eat more with sweetener than without it!" Nevertheless, there are more than six thousand foods in the United States alone that contain sweeteners. It is no wonder that the United States is facing an epidemic of obesity. In Europe, too, we are no longer far from it.

Psychological as well as physiological aspects play a role. Anyone who drinks a Diet Coke (or comparable "light," so-called reduced-sugar drinks), "indulges" in something sweet afterward because the brain is not satisfied with the sweetener and sends signals that drive it to consume more sugar.

The use of sweeteners by women during pregnancy is also said to cause children to become overweight in their first year of life (the disposition for the associated diseases would thus practically begin "in the cradle").

However, in addition to the general weight gain due to (excessive) sugar consumption, the risks for abdominal obesity (the accumulation of fat in the abdominal region, which in turn is a risk factor for certain diseases), metabolic syndrome (one of the most important risk factors for cardiovascular disease), cardiovascular diseases, type 2 diabetes, as well as high blood pressure and strokes also increase.

3.7.2 Sugar Substitutes and Their Effect: The Health Consequences of Sweet Indulgence

Some sweeteners even have the reputation of directly promoting cancer. One such sweetener is the widely used aspartame (with the abbreviation E 951 as a food additive permitted by the authorities), which is found in many "light" products, soft drinks, chewing gum, and even in over five hundred different medications.

Aspartame is two hundred times sweeter than sugar, but loses its sweetness when heated and therefore cannot be used in baking or cooking. In our bodies, it is converted into poisonous methanol, among other things.

According to an Israeli study, the sugar substitutes saccharin (E 954), sucralose (E 955), and aspartame (E 951) induced changes in the intestinal flora, which had an unfavorable effect on blood sugar levels and promoted metabolic diseases.

The Italian scientist Morando Soffritti, director of the European Institute of Oncology and Environmental Science in Bologna, who has published over 150 scientific studies, has been fighting for many years for a reassessment of the dangers of aspartame by the health and food authorities and expressly warns about aspartame as a carcinogen: so far in vain!

Despite a convincing number of studies on the health-damaging or carcinogenic effects of aspartame, the manufacturers of aspartame and the related "experts" and authorities keep dismissing all concerns and continue to sell their chemicals, which are permitted as food additives, without scruples, while the number of chronically ill people keeps growing.

Among the sugar substitutes or sweeteners that we classify as dangerous to our health, but which are permitted additives under food law, are
acesulfame-K and sodium cyclamate, in addition to the already mentioned
substitutes saccharin, sucralose, and aspartame. Acesulfame-K (E 950) is a
synthetic substance that has also been linked to the development of cancer.

Sodium cyclamate (E 952) does not cause insulin secretion and is heat stable. It has been banned in the United States since 1969, but is still permitted
in Germany. In animal experiments, a damaging effect on testicles and sperm
could be proven.

Saccharin (E 954) is one of the oldest synthetic sweeteners, used for the
first time one hundred years ago for people with diabetes. It is suspected
to raise blood sugar levels and have a harmful effect on the intestinal flora.
In Canada saccharin is banned. Sucralose (E 955) is made from table sugar
using chlorine. Sucralose is suspected of triggering irritable bowel syndrome and of significantly reducing good intestinal bacteria, which not only
has an unfavorable effect on the blood sugar level, but can also damage the
intestine in general.

3.7.3 The Sugar Alcohols

Sugar alcohols are found in small amounts in plants, but are produced syn-
thetically on a large scale for human consumption from wood or plant fibers.
They are therefore not natural products in the strict sense. Compared to the
sweeteners mentioned above, however, they are all much less harmful to our
health. If they are consumed in large quantities, they often cause flatulence,
cramps, or diarrhea.

As with all sugar substitutes, sugar alcohols can tempt you to miss out on
a healthy, conscious and natural diet: They keep the craving for sweetness
alive and tempt you to unhealthy eating habits. Used in moderation, however, they can add an enjoyable taste to food. And enjoyment is also part of
a fulfilled life!

Isomalt (E 953), a mixture of two sugar alcohols, is suitable for a ketogenic
diet, as are xylitol (E 967), which is made from corn cob residues, or beech
or birch wood, and erythritol (E 968), which is made from table sugar with

the help of a special fungus. They do not affect insulin levels and can also be used for cooking. Of these, erythritol seems to us to be the most suitable sugar alcohol as a substitute or replacement because it causes less diarrhea and flatulence, has fewer calories than isomalt, and does not have the "cool" taste of xylitol. Mannitol (E 421) and sorbitol (E 420) complete the list of sugar alcohols, without adding any special properties.

Stevia and Steviol Glycosides

Stevia is a perennial plant from South America, also called sweet leaf or honey herb, whose dried leaves are used by the South American population for sweetening. This herb is thirty to forty-five times sweeter than sugar.

The steviol glycosides (E 960) extracted from stevia have been approved as a sweetener in the European Union since 2011, but organic foods are not allowed to contain steviol glycosides.

In addition to its sweetening power, which is two hundred to four hundred times greater than that of table sugar, it has a licorice-like, slightly bitter taste. Therefore, stevia is best combined with a sugar alcohol, for example, erythritol. Concerns that stevia would have a damaging effect on the genetic makeup of humans could not be confirmed. Even when administered in very high doses, animal experiments did not show any noticeable side effects, which can be said of very few sweeteners. However, a certain maximum amount (which is quickly reached due to the enormous sweetening power of stevia) should not be exceeded here either, in order not to harm the organism.

Honey

Honey is a gift from nature and a real raw food product. It consists of up to 80 percent glucose and fructose in roughly equal parts; the remaining 20 percent is water. The exact composition can vary somewhat depending on the type of honey.

Honey also contains small amounts of vitamins (for example, vitamin C, thiamine, riboflavin, and niacin), enzymes, and amino acids, but also minerals (such as calcium, potassium, sodium, and chlorine) and trace elements (such as iron, zinc, and copper). In total, it contains up to 245 different natural substances, which are also antibacterial, antifungal, antioxidant, and anti-inflammatory. Although the sugars in honey can cause more tooth decay than normal brown or table sugar (among other things, honey also sticks to the teeth more strongly), it is much healthier than normal sugar for the reasons mentioned above.

Honey should never be heated above 40°C (104°F), because it loses its natural antibiotic effect and many of its ingredients are destroyed. The healing effect of honey has been known and appreciated for thousands of years. For gastrointestinal inflammation or diarrhea, externally for inflammations of the skin or fungal infections, honey is an effective natural remedy without side effects.

It can also be used as a prebiotic to nourish our intestinal flora and renders the fungal toxins from mold—called aflatoxins—harmless.

However, babies of up to twelve months of age should not consume honey, because the spores of the clostridia bacteria that may be present in honey cannot be destroyed by babies' immature intestinal flora and can germinate in the babies' intestines and develop into active bacteria. Their neurotoxin can lead to internal poisoning and even paralysis. For children over a year old and adults, these bacteria are not a problem, because the microbiome is developed enough to be able to destroy harmful germs. Depending on the origin and processing method (honey should not actually be processed!), many commercially available honeys are mixed together, heated, or stretched with water and sugar to make the product appear "even" and quite simply to increase the quantity (and profit). Therefore, when buying, always look for the best quality and the seal of approval of the beekeepers' association.

GOOD—BUT RIGHT

As always, it is the quantity that determines whether a food is healthy or at all harmful to our health. Enjoy organic honey in moderation and do not use it in baking or hot drinks. Allow tea to cool to below 40°C (104°F) before adding honey to it, and be conscious of the quantities you use. A teaspoon of honey is a remedy; too much of a good thing, like too much sugar, has a detrimental effect and the healing power is lost.

Avoid synthetic sweeteners in all forms. They are potentially toxic and probably carcinogenic according to our twelve-part understanding of risk.

Use sugar alcohols, preferably erythritol, only in moderation and enjoy with awareness! Use stevia only in small quantities if its typical taste appeals to you, preferably mixed with a pinch of erythritol. Use bee honey in moderation and do not overheat it.

3.8 The Shift of the Immune System

Psyche and body are closely connected. Our personality blossoms only when both are harmoniously intertwined. The following looks at the authenticity of the reader and the shadow that is cast over life when the immune system is out of sync.

One of the strangest phenomena of the immunological response around a cancerous tumor is the shifting of the immune system of the host organism around it. A functioning immune system can recognize cancer cells and break them down effectively, every day. However, if a proliferation of cancer cells has been able to develop into a manifest tumor, we have to admit that the immune system was overtaxed in its defensive function and could no longer protect us sufficiently. The further successful spread of cancer cells to a manifest tumor is increasingly accompanied with a totally altered immune function. After some time, part of the immune system even begins to protect the tumor. Figuratively speaking, the immune system has confusedly lost sight of the essentials and its actual tasks and works against the organism in favor of the cancer cells. But how is this possible? And what can we do about it?

————

On the biological level, it is above all inflammation and the associated lack of oxygen as well as an increasing overacidification of the microenvironment around the tumor that provide the fuel for this immunological misfortune or cause the reversal of the behavior of the immune cells.

For some years, immunologists have distinguished two types of immune cells that play an important role in this. They are both called macrophages, which means *big eater* or *scavenger cell*, and are divided into M1 and M2 macrophages, among others. M1 macrophages are referred to as *classically activated* and ensure inflammation and a positive, anticancer immune response. M2 macrophages are *alternatively activated* and bring about tumor spread and inhibition of the immune control of cancer. M2 macrophages thus work for the cancer colony and against the host organism. M1 can transform into M2.

What makes this possible? And what is the point? Anyone who reads immunological literature on the subject runs the risk of drowning in literally hundreds of details. Moreover, the biochemical "maps" that describe this terrain change every year, and it happens at every new symposium that experts report on the "latest state of the error" (German: "neueste[n] Stand des Irrtums"), as it is sometimes humorously referred to among experts. Inflammatory processes and lack of oxygen, infections, and toxins seem to play the most important roles in this change from M1 to M2, although the details are very complex and sometimes contradictory. The question is: Who or what is controlling all of this? The already mentioned topic (see the introduction) of how the mind relates to matter, also emerges very clearly here. When the immunologist says that the protein interferon-gamma stimulates the macrophages to transform themselves into M1 macrophages and the protein interleukin-4, which is produced by T-helper cells (special immune cells), stimulates the transformation into M2 macrophages, then this is not the answer to the basic question, but rather a shifting of this question into ever smaller biochemical details. Just as the notes made of ink on musical score sheets do not control the orchestra musicians, but are read, interpreted, and conducted to the members of the orchestra by the conductor, proteins control life! It is almost palpable that life is not controlled by substances, but by energy, which manifests itself in the body as electromagnetic transmissions of force and then in chemical substances and their interactions. Who really controls our life? What is the "conductor" called?

Let us look at the function of the immune system for our life from another, perhaps higher perspective than from the purely biological level.

3.8.1 "Blood Is a Very Special Juice": The Immune System and the Ego Function

In Goethe's *Faust*, the main character of the epochal drama (which Goethe worked on in successive versions from 1772 to 1832), Doctor Faust, makes a pact with Mephisto (the devil) effective by using a drop of blood as his signature.

This makes it clear, as in many fairy tales and myths, that our blood is in a special way an expression of our distinctive inner being. It is likely that blood has been regarded as a carrier of life force since the beginning of mankind. If a human being or animal bleeds to death, its life force also dwindles, until he or she dies. For this reason, blood has always been regarded as the secret of the origin of life, the color red as the color of fertility. The motif of blood, the drop of blood, signing with blood, or sealing a pact with blood can be found in the mythology of various peoples and in countless fairy tales. Also the drinking of blood in order to absorb the life force of the being from which it comes is mythologically charged. But this was also a widespread practice in Germany until a few decades ago: Besides the idea that nothing should perish or go unused, blood soup or blood sausage were dishes after slaughter.

In many religions, too, blood has a similar symbolism as an expression of life: It is the essence of the personality of its bearer; it stands, so to speak, for the "self." Because life is given by God, blood is therefore sacred and may not be consumed in some religions: in Judaism, for example, neither in profane life nor during a religious sacrifice. In the Christian Eucharist of the Lord's Supper, the symbolic ingestion of wine as the *blood* of the Redeemer is the center of religious activity.

In the blood, we also find the predominant number of our immune cells, the white blood cells. They circulate through our entire organism every moment of our lives to seek out and ward off intruders, be they microorganisms or cells that are foreign to us, such as cancer cells. As long as this constant defense against the foreign, against the *not-me*, functions in our bodies, we are healthy. If this mechanism is thrown out of kilter, we become ill. If there is a shift in the defense of our physical self, we either get an autoimmune disease or, if we do not recognize cells that have become foreign to us, we get cancer. If our immune system even protects the foreign cells, the distress is at its greatest: A cancer can now spread within us, completely unchecked.

———

In the psychospiritual realm of our consciousness, the self is thus connected with the distinction between me and the world around me. In psychiatric illnesses, for example in psychosis, the clear distinction between my thoughts and the thoughts of others is lost. Foreign thoughts impose themselves and begin to live in the consciousness of the ill person in a strange, psychotic way. The healthy boundaries between subject and object blur and merge, and chaos ensues. In the case of cancer, this plays out in the physical body. What is interesting in the chosen example is that there is scientific evidence that psychoses and cancers avoid each other. Either the pathological shift occurs only in consciousness (psychosis, schizophrenia) or in the physical (cancer), apparently rarely in both areas at the same time.

Who am I? This is a question you can contemplate for your whole life. As a doctor, I have come to the following understanding of the "self" of my patient: Their self is that which constantly, throughout life, preserves and delimits itself from everything that is not the self. It is something that is separated from the whole world, something entirely its own, and yet is meaningfully connected to the world and belongs to it. This is as true of biological life as it is of psychological life. The self is the guardian of the boundary between the world and that part of the world that is entirely its own, namely my own. Physically, or even biologically manifested, we find this function realized in the form of our immune system.

It is not always the case that we are in a balanced center with the focus on our consciousness, our behavior, and our feelings. Balance is a pendulum: at one time self-centered on our needs, at another time concerned about our environment and fellow human beings. If, instead of being a healthy pendulum, our inner alignment consciously or unconsciously slips into one-sidedness and the *spiritual swinging back* no longer takes place, sooner or later our health will also be affected. Deviations from the *oscillating balance* that we call health, can be, for example, the following extremes:

When I feel responsible for too many things and my self-boundary becomes too wide. I allow the world to get too close to me and cannot separate myself from it enough.

When I feel responsible for too little and my boundary with the world is too closed, sealed off, and my ego remains too selectively related to itself. Then I am hardly interested in the world around me and I am interested mainly in myself. Pathological forms of this one-sidedness are unhealthy narcissism—including narcissistic personality disorder—or antisocial (dissocial) personality disorder.

Personally, cancer seems to me to be a physical *counterbalance* for a too weak boundary between me and the world. Many of my patients describe the perception of feeling responsible for everything and not being able to separate themselves.

The "essence" of a cancerous tumor is quite simple to understand: It cares only about itself, like a frightened deserter, who realizes that his army can no longer win the war. Like someone or something who steps out of the gears of an aspiration that is no longer achievable, like something that has no perception for other beings. Cancer seems like a representative of a primal form of mere survival. Is there is a gesture in it or even a message for the sufferers? Does it show me what I should do?

Within this approach, inflammation shows itself as a self-force in its "fiery" way to regain the lost integrity. In latent or chronic inflammation (silent inflammation), however, this force is in an ineffective continuous struggle and exhausts itself. The area to be repaired becomes a wound that—instead of healing—is only nurtured. In this chronic weakness, cancer finally develops, which is then nurtured, instead of the wound, by the immune system: A new type of immune cell is formed, the M2 macrophages, which wrap themselves around the cancer like a protective shield and nurse it like a wound so that the other immune cells do not attack it.

3.8.2 The Transition to Psychoneuroimmunology

So if we look for the control of the life processes of the immune system in our consciousness, a special aspect of psychoneuroimmunology arises: *consciousness medicine*.

However, our consciousness is itself of a very complex nature, and there is not just one consciousness in us, but many. The different levels of consciousness represent different degrees of consciousness or unconsciousness. A simplified classification initially reveals three levels:

1. The deep subconscious: This is connected to the basal sections of our brain, the brain stem, which is also the oldest part of our brain in terms of development. This is where the most elementary regulatory processes take place, controlling our blood pressure, heart rate,

breathing, and important reflexes such as eyelid closure, swallowing, and coughing reflexes.

2. Semiconscious consciousness: This describes the indeterminate feelings from dreaming to clearly defined and conscious feelings. This range is assigned to the neurological area of the diencephalon, the limbic system. This is where the neurological roots of our emotional and instinctive behavior lie. Fear, desire, even our unconscious, constant search reflex (the search reflex attracts our attention and occurs as soon as something moves in our field of vision, which is, among other things, one of the central driving forces of all computer games), as well as anger and desire are mirrored neurologically here.

3. And finally, we have the fully conscious consciousness, which is evident in the clear, conscious thinking or in the mindset of *mindfulness*. The neurological area of the frontal brain corresponds to this, which distinguishes the human brain from its animal ancestors.

———————

The conflict of the out-of-balance immune system, which maintains too many inflammations and can no longer take care of the life-threatening cancer cells, is confronted with another conflict or several conflicts on the level of consciousness. The individual partial aspects of the tasks that life sets you, and the associated demands that are perceived in consciousness, can sometimes no longer be reconciled with each other due to inner conflicts. The mental force field of consciousness loses its coherence when, for example, I want to do something, but I don't feel good about it, that is, the ability to be coherent and work best in one direction.

The immune system that is out of balance, maintains too much inflammation, and takes care of life-threatening cancer cells is in a kind of *inner* conflict of its own: It can no longer work coherently—meaningfully in one direction—in order to serve the higher organism. It splits forces and energies, thereby blocking itself or the whole self-healing system, and through this conflict contributes to the self-destruction of the entire organism.

Accordingly, the incoherent consciousness with activities going in different directions, blocking each other, is caught in a permanent inner conflict and can no more solve the problems of semiconsciousness, the subconscious, or other repressed conflicts, in the same way that the immune system, led astray, can no longer recognize and break down the cancer cells.

Just as it is biologically important to expose the overloaded sites of an insidious inflammation and to reverse its milieu, it is important to uncover inner conflicts so that they can be resolved. The feelings of shame, guilt, fear, disappointment, or inner paralysis must first come to consciousness before they can be transformed, guided by therapeutic experience, into acceptance, courage, and genuine, healthy self-love. As mentioned elsewhere, fever therapy can be of enormous benefit to both healing responses. When experiencing a fever, the body converts smoldering inflammation temporarily and in a controlled way into an acute fever response, and then shuts it down completely into freedom from inflammation.

The soul goes through a healing crisis in a fever and thus experiences feelings much more strongly and is able to express them in order to let them go afterward. This healing crisis can be observed in milder illnesses—even without a fever—and is the reason why, for example, we feel miserable, vulnerable, sore, and open to attack even during a mere cold. Thoughts and feelings seem heavy and dark, but clear up as we recover.

In the Arcadia practice, we offer our patients coloring pencils and a drawing pad before and after whole-body hyperthermia (fever therapy) to illustrate their mood (see chapter 5). Following the therapy, the calm mood of the pictures as a mirror or possible expression for the clarification of inner conflicts can be observed again and again and is an amazing phenomenon.

In this sense, coherence is the state in which the different cells of the body and especially of the immune system support the whole organism, that is, body and life. Coherence is also the state in which the different parts of the brain—the unconscious volitional processes of the brain stem, the feelings of the diencephalon, and the thoughts and principles of the frontal brain—serve the same goal: the personal life design, the conception of one's own life plan, and the realization and development of one's own personality.

It is therefore incoherent—lacking congruence—to do something different, something that does not feel good and right, not doing or being able to do something that is actually wanted, to want something that is not allowed or socially accepted.

Against the backdrop of the holistic understanding of the human presented here, it seems to me personally to be of utmost importance to keep in mind the coherence for both our consciousness and our biological physicality in all healing efforts and to recognize that both systems work hand in hand and that recovery and health can take place only in mutual agreement. Inner conflicts must therefore be resolved and transformed in the same way that material toxins must be eliminated from the organism and chronic inflammation must be healed. If coherence is lost—both in the psychoemotional and in the immunological processes—this promotes the development of cancer and the uninhibited growth of cancer tumors.

The therapeutic goal is therefore to bring the immune system back into balance and to establish coherence so that the immune system can specifically serve life and health, and in consciousness the areas of feeling, thinking, understanding, planning, and active wanting can be (re)aligned with what serves the true meaning of life and the creative expression of the personality.

3.8.3 Healing Meditations: Aligning Consciousness and Promoting Coherence

In the sense of consciousness medicine, affirmations or meditations can be used to increase coherence in the inner field of force. The following text is a suggestion of how this can be implemented. Try it out.

- Sit comfortably and preferably upright on a chair. For these exercises, it is helpful to place your arms relaxed on your lap and not to cross your legs, so that the energy can flow freely, you can relax, and your breathing becomes deep.
- Read the following text slowly, for example, one line on an exhale.
- Take a short break during the inhale and read the next line again on the exhale.
- The slower you can read this text without breaking your train of thought, the deeper the effect of the exercise on your inner coherence.

- You can also recite these or other meditation texts to yourself on a dictation machine, which is already available on every smartphone these days.
- Speak slowly and deliberately, then the meditation will have an optimal coherence-increasing effect on the various areas of your brain and thus have a positive effect on your self-healing powers.
- After a few practice attempts, you can begin to lengthen the intervals between the lines and slow down the flow of consciousness.
- When disturbing thoughts arise, imagine—as in other meditations—that these thoughts are clouds in the sky that are passing by and that you can calmly observe and allow to pass. Simply direct your attention to the meditation text again and again, and let go of the disturbing thoughts again and again without evaluating them.

The effect of such a meditation exercise starts first in the consciousness and spreads, the longer you work with it, to your psychoemotional level. Finally, after some practice, the effect also reaches the biological level and thus influences immunological control processes. During the exercises it is helpful to feel the content of the meditation. First of all, the individual words, the lines, and gradually the whole meditation.

But how does one do this? Firstly, by slowly letting the words *drift through the soul*—similar to the clouds mentioned above, that is, without pressure, without evaluating them, without wanting too much, slowly and deliberately—and then also through repetition. In hypnotherapy, since Milton Erikson at the latest, a "healing trance" has been discussed, which comes about through the slow repetition of desired thought content and messages. From the intellectual understanding, which usually arises immediately during reading, a feeling gradually develops. By generating this new feeling ("I feel my health forces becoming strong in me again. . . . I feel myself healing."), you gradually send more and more effective biochemical messengers to your immune system, which is now more coherent with your life again and protects and heals you.

Since the healing meditations discussed here can also be used and are effective in other contexts, in line with our holistic world view, we have decided to describe them in chapter 6. There you will find a compilation of the instructions for the healing meditations mentioned here and you can also apply them in relation to other chapters and content.

3.9 Mitochondria: Power Plants of the Cells

From primeval single-cell organisms to differentiated cellular symbiosis and the *energy-saving program* of cell metabolism as primeval heritage, mitochondria are small cell organelles (structures within a cell with specific functions), which are also commonly regarded as the *power plants of the cells*.

With their help, energy is produced from fats and carbohydrates, which all the cells in our body need for all their life-supporting and life-sustaining processes of formation and degradation.

Up until about two billion years ago, mitochondria were independent bacteria that joined forces with cells of higher life forms in the course of evolution. This endosymbiont theory is now considered scientifically proven—that they are the descendants of archaebacteria that were taken up by single-cell organisms (protocytes) in primeval times and have lived together with them ever since, forming a functional unit. In exchange for a protected living environment, they provided and continue to provide energy for all life processes. This community of life was the prerequisite for all higher life on our planet, from primitive animals to humans. Our cells thus live in symbiosis with the descendants of primordial bacteria (archaebacteria).

This is an interesting fact when we also look at the connection between mitochondria and cancer in the following: The ancient, *bacterial* heritage of mitochondria is for this reason the possession of its own DNA and, in addition to a special *form of behavior* that we will discuss later, the property of dividing every four to five days, as other bacteria do.

3.9.1 Structure and Function of the Cellular Power Plants

Mitochondria are so small that they can hardly be identified with a light microscope. They are two to five micrometers long and half a micrometer to two micrometers in diameter. The greater the energy requirement of a cell and the more metabolic activity takes place in it, the more mitochondria we find in it. Red blood cells contain no mitochondria, blood platelets contain two to six, nerve cells contain about ten thousand, and an egg cell contains up to several hundred thousand mitochondria in its cell plasma. The mitochondria of the heart muscle even make up 36 percent of the total weight of the heart!

Mitochondria have a smooth surface and a complex folded inner double membrane (cell skin). This organelle, an organ of a cell, is bounded by the outer membrane, while the second skin, which is everted inward, forms folds and fans. Enclosed by it is the fluid mitochondrial matrix inside the mitochondrion, in which the DNA as well as ribosomes (protein-forming corpuscles) and small vesicles (filled with fluid) float.

The DNA (deoxyribonucleic acid) carries the genetic material of the mitochondrion, and proteins are produced at the ribosomes, while very different processes take place in the vesicles. They are also responsible for the transport of many substances into the cell.

Due to the folding of the inner membrane, one gram of liver tissue has an inner surface of about three square meters, where the energy carriers of the entire cell metabolism, the energy-carrying ATP molecules, are formed (see figure 3.3). The sum of the highly complex biochemical reactions that lead to the production of ATP is called the respiratory chain: Energy in the form of phosphorous molecules (ADP and ATP), which are needed for almost all tasks of cellular life, is produced from carbohydrates and fats during glycolysis (sugar splitting) or the oxidation of fatty acids, with the consumption of oxygen.

More precisely, it is glucose, specifically dextrose, that the cells need from carbohydrates so that life energy can be produced. During the digestion process, the

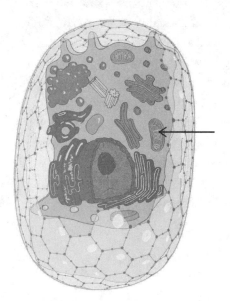

Figure 3.3. Cell with its mitochondria (arrow) and the inner mitochondrial cell membrane, folded in a complex manner, in cross-section.

carbohydrates from cereals, vegetable, or legumes, for example, are broken down into glucose, and some energy is already released outside the mitochondria during the glycolysis. During this process of glycolysis, a substance called pyruvate (pyruvic acid) is produced, which can now be introduced into the mitochondria, where it sets in motion the essential part of energy production. This process is called the citrate cycle. A lot of B vitamins are needed for this, but also many micronutrients, such as zinc, manganese, iron, copper, and CoQ10. The crucial factor in this process is that it involves the generation of energy using oxygen. It is at the same time much more efficient and produces eighteen times more ATP per glucose molecule than glycolysis without oxygen is capable of.

During this energy production, a constant building up and breaking down of electrical charges occurs on the mitochondrial membrane, called electron potentials, by building up chemical imbalances. Protons diffuse from the positively charged inner space into the space with the negative membrane charge and the lower proton concentration. Protons, neutrons, and electrons belong to the building blocks of atoms, of which all matter is composed. Electrons are the smallest energy carriers that, in modern physics, represent the massless transition between matter and nonmatter, energy and light.

Do we find here the modern correlate of the life force known from antiquity and the Asian healing arts, the chi or prana? The high mitochondrial density in the heart also corresponds to the ancient concept of the heart as the seat of life. Could precisely this highly complex process also be a possible explanation for the phenomenon of the living luminescence, as described in chapter 2? Energy is also needed for the natural death (apoptosis) of the cell to make room for a new generation of cells. Like the entire body, which is constantly being built up and broken down, mitochondria also live in a perpetual process of multiplying, consuming, growing, or breaking down.

In his aphorism "Nature: Fragment from the Journal of Tiefurt" (1783), Goethe already described this necessity of dying in order to "have a lot of life." He wrote: "Nature! We are surrounded and embraced by it. . . . Life is its most beautiful invention, and death is its artifice in order to have a lot of life."

However, cancer cells have lost this ability to die. One could also say that due to their heritage, as described above, they are able to evade symbiotic coexistence within a whole organism by becoming autonomous "lone fighters." While intact cells die off when it is time, for the benefit for the organism as a whole, cancer cells go into the primitive state in which they can gain energy even without oxygen—ideally from sugar. One of the main goals of modern cancer therapy and the task of numerous anticancer drugs is therefore to revive apoptosis and to set natural death in motion again.

3.9.2 The Anaerobic Fermentation of Carbohydrates

But what happens when cells develop into cancer cells by becoming autonomous and coming out of a symbiotic cell association? When we work hard physically, when we exercise extensively or do sports, certain cells in the body—depending on what we are doing or which muscles we are particularly straining—have a very high energy demand for a short time. The glycolysis described above produces more pyruvate than the mitochondria can absorb.

At this point, the cellular power plants switch from energy production with the help of oxygen to one that can still provide some energy without oxygen: anaerobic energy production, which still produces two molecules of ATP per glucose molecule instead of the thirty-two molecules of ATP from glycolysis with oxygen (aerobic). Because there is too little oxygen available due to acute exertion, the excess pyruvate is now fermented into lactic acid under anaerobic (oxygen-free) conditions, and lactate is formed.

If this kind of exertion happens occasionally and is followed by a recovery phase, the body can completely break down the pyruvate lactate that has formed.

If, for example, we have overdone it a bit during exercise, perhaps because we are unfit or out of practice, lactic acid is the deposit product that gives us noticeable muscle aches.

If we look at the positive side of this *cell heritage* and look at situations in the past, our ancestors were able to cope with unforeseen or untrained exertion, for example, when they had to flee from a bear or suddenly had to defend themselves. Without anaerobic glycolysis, they would have been out of breath pretty quickly. Fortunately, today it is less often a matter of self-defense; much more often it is a sprint to the train station or the sport being practiced.

However, today we have an overabundance of carbohydrates in our diet and a simultaneous lack of exercise. Too few micronutrients and too many environmental toxins or too much psychological stress also lead to a permanent or excessive production of lactic acid, just like permanent physical overload, for example, what we would see in competitive sports.

So our modern life has created many other threats for us to which our mitochondria react. Toxins, side effects of medicines such as cholesterol-reducing statin drugs, lack of exercise and oxygen, and an unhealthy diet are such risk factors. Researchers now believe that neurodegenerative diseases—such as Alzheimer's disease, multiple sclerosis, amyotrophic lateral sclerosis, and Parkinson's disease—diabetes mellitus, cancer, cardiovascular diseases, and obesity are diseases that can be significantly promoted or even caused by mitochondrial damage.

The first visible and noticeable sign of this permanent overproduction of lactate is the fatigue of body and mind. Listlessness and a lack of drive also increase (for example, in depression), as does susceptibility to infections due to the compromised immune system.

One of the best-known scientists who describes cancer as a metabolic disease is the American doctor and professor Thomas N. Seyfried. His book *Cancer as a Metabolic Disease* is the groundbreaking standard work on this subject, in which he continues the legacy of Otto Warburg, among others, and shows that complex changes in the oxygen, sugar, and mitochondrial metabolism ultimately lead to cancer.

———

However, mitochondria also react sensitively to oxidative stress, the free radicals. These include the oxygen radicals that are formed in the mitochondria during inflammations—for example, with arthritis and allergies—or infections, with an unbalanced diet and nicotine, drug, and excessive alcohol consumption. But also after operations and injuries, due to medication (for example, cytostatics), pesticides, and environmental toxins (for example, lead, cadmium, mercury, ozone, smog, radioactive or ionizing radiation, extended exposure to television or computer screens, mobile phones, UV rays, and so forth), an excessive number of free radicals are produced. Physical or mental stress also releases massive amounts of free radicals through the breakdown of stress hormones. Because they actually work for the immune system and are supposed to act against foreign organisms, but due to our current lifestyle the unfavorable effects on the mitochondria are often too high or too varied or simply permanent, the organism cannot sufficiently ward off the excessive free radicals and becomes damaged itself. If inflammation becomes chronic or toxins cannot be sufficiently broken down, the energy production in the mitochondria of a cell permanently decreases.

As a result, signals are sent to the cell nucleus, which then activates an emergency program for the cell's survival. It goes into the old primitive state, in which it can survive even without oxygen and preferably only with sugar as fuel, and becomes a cancer cell.

In his book, *Mitochondria: More Life Energy Due to Healthy Cellular Power Plants*, Christian Dittrich-Opitz describes the vicious circle that can then set in, "as the self-destruction process is driven forward ever faster by glucose-induced free radicals." There is no energy left to die off *in time* to make room for the new, healthier cells in the organism as a whole. The cell thus becomes an "autistic deserter." As a single cell, it looks after only its own interests from this point on. It has left the cell association, the syncytium, to fend for itself.

Per sugar molecule (glucose), such a cell at this point produces only the said two instead of the other thirty-eight molecules of ATP, that a healthy cell can produce under aerobic combustion, through anaerobic fermentation. However, this amount is not sufficient to carry out all mature cell functions. But it is enough for survival as a single-cell organism, and that is what matters to it.

3.9.3 **Mitochondria and Age**

Irreparable damage to the mitochondria naturally increases with age, and the body's ability to produce energy as effectively as possible becomes more and more impaired. But the mitochondria themselves also age. For them, obtaining ATP through the glycolysis of carbohydrates is energetically easier than obtaining ATP through the oxidation of fatty acids. However, glucose combustion generally produces more free radicals, which accelerate the aging process of the mitochondria. But aging mitochondria rely more and more on glucose for energy because the mitochondria gradually lose the ability to burn fatty acids effectively. Habituation and age can result in dependence on sugar or carbohydrates and growing fat deposits. So far, it has not been conclusively clarified whether the increasing aging of the mitochondria or their damage is the cause or simply a phenomenon for the aging process of the entire organism.

Treatments and Supplements that Activate Mitochondria

ORTHOMOLECULAR MEDICINE

Orthomolecular medicine includes the administration of vitamins, minerals, and trace elements, sometimes in high doses. The term was introduced in 1968 by Linus Pauling (1901–1994), American Nobel Peace Prize and Chemistry laureate, and is composed of the Greek word *orthos* (meaning "correct") and the Latin word *molecule* (meaning "small mass"). *Molecular* thus stands for the "simplest form describing a substance." From the point of view of orthomolecular medicine, an existing imbalance in the body creates the prerequisite for diseases. The targeted use of minerals, trace elements, and vitamins in special dosages is not only intended to cure diseases, but also to prevent them and serves, for example, to optimize the metabolism and activate detoxification.

INTERMITTENT HYPOXIA–HYPEROXIA THERAPY (IHHT)

IHHT is a special inhalation therapy that particularly accelerates the stimulation of mitochondrial renewal and the necessary death of old, damaged mitochondria. In this process, an air-oxygen mixture with a higher O_2 concentration is first offered at intervals of a few minutes, and then a low air-O_2 mixture is administered for a few minutes. This alternation of hyperoxia (too much O_2) and hypoxia (too little O_2) stimulates the death of damaged, old mitochondria in our body and simultaneously promotes the creation of new mitochondria.

DICHLOROACETIC ACID

Dichloroacetic acid is a substance that can at least partially repair the mitochondrial metabolism. It has been studied for decades in numerous scientific studies as a potent anticancer agent and has been shown to be effective. Unfortunately, such agents remain stuck in oncological research at a lower study phase, for which there is a lack of funds for further clinical research or because there is no lobby available for it due to the low prospect of profit and patentability.

ALPHA LIPOIC ACID

Alpha lipoic acid reduces oxidative damage by binding free oxygen radicals, thus preventing nerve damage. It is also considered by scientists to be the *most powerful* antioxidant that can slow down the aging process.

PYRROLOQUINOLINE QUINONE

In the case of pyrroloquinoline quinone, PQQ for short, it is still unclear whether it can be classified as a vitamin and assigned to the B vitamins. PQQ is said to have a growth- and metabolism-stimulating effect on mitochondria.

COENZYME Q10

CoQ10 is a component of mitochondria and is produced by the body itself, but production can decline with age. This coenzyme plays an important role in the defense against oxidative stress by capturing free radicals. It is significantly involved in energy metabolism.

RESVERATROL

Resveratrol is an active ingredient in red wine that can suppress even minor inflammatory reactions in an anti-inflammatory manner and is effective against free radicals. Life-prolonging effects and positive reactions of the mitochondria could be observed through the administration of resveratrol. The concentrations that are necessary for this can best be achieved by the administration of supplements. The well-dosed consumption of dry red wine, which is about 250 milliliters per day for men and about 150 milliliters per day for women, has been shown in many studies to have a positive effect on the risk of cardiovascular disease and cancer. However, it is important to

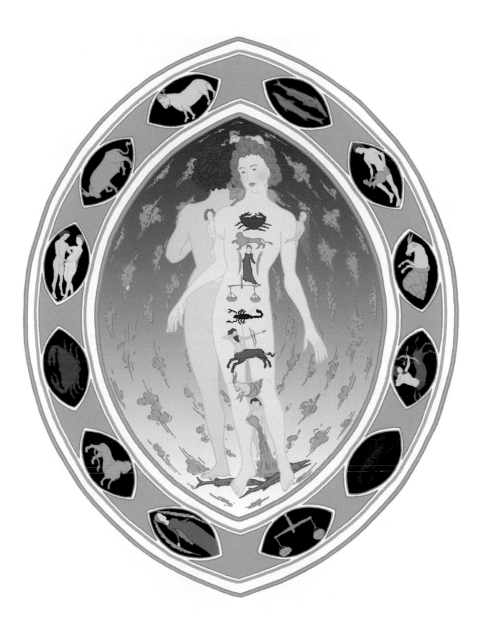

Figure 1. *L'homme anatomique*, or anatomical man, as he is integrated into the forces of the cosmos, as featured in the book illumination *Les Très Riches Heures du Duc de Berry* by the "Limbourg Brothers." This late-medieval masterpiece shows us that holism was the rule, not the exception, in human understanding of health and disease.

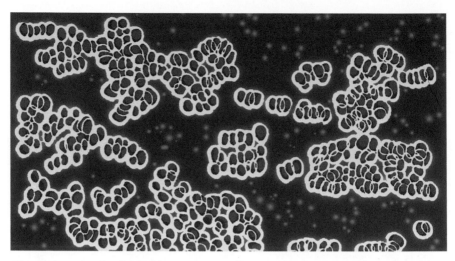

Figure 2. Unstained blood, 400x magnification in the dark-field microscope, strongly agglutinated red blood cells, which form rouleaux, before treatment with PEMF. Agglutinated blood cells can perform only a fraction of the oxygen–carbon dioxide exchange compared to freely moving blood cells.

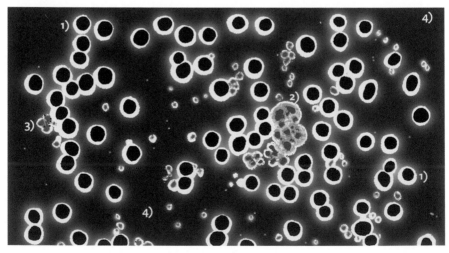

Figure 3. Unstained blood, 400x magnification in the dark-field microscope, immediately after a twenty-minute treatment with PEMF:
1 Red blood cells (erythrocytes): transport of oxygen and carbon dioxide
2 White blood cells (leukocytes): represent part of our immune system
3 Platelets (thrombocytes): contribute to blood clotting
4 Invisible, black background: the blood plasma with its dissolved proteins and salts

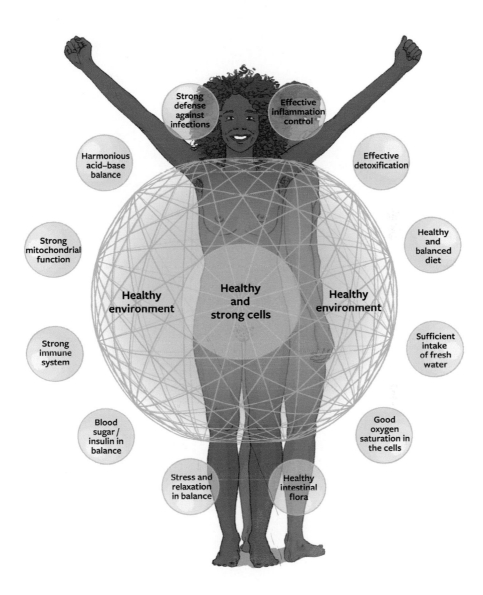

Figure 4. The vital field with its twelve elements represents the human being in the midst of a network of relationships in which each of the twelve factors can be influenced and modulated by the others. Through this constant exchange, the continuous building up and breaking down processes and their positive influence, we are able to promote, strengthen, and maintain health.

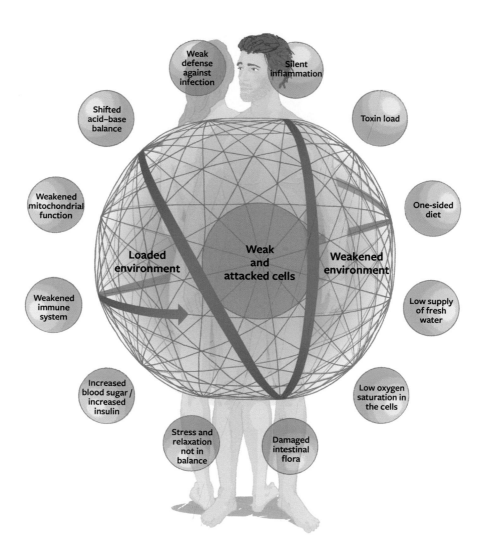

Figure 5. Factors of the vital field that are out of balance can be positively influenced, while "tilted" fields can be brought back into balance to revive self-healing powers and strengthen the entire organism.

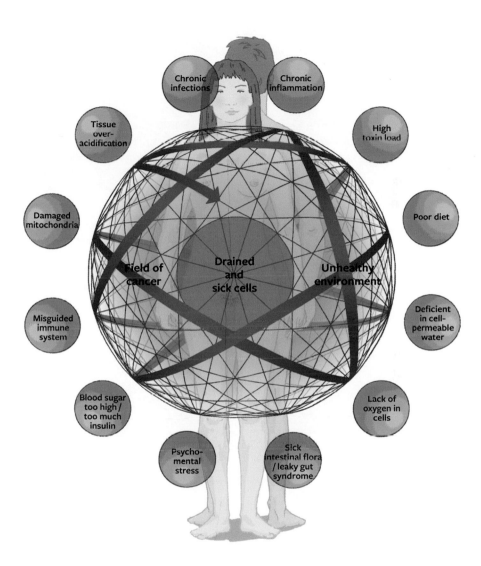

Figure 6. If too many of the areas that affect our mental and physical health remain permanently imbalanced, this creates an unhealthy environment in which diseases like cancer can develop.

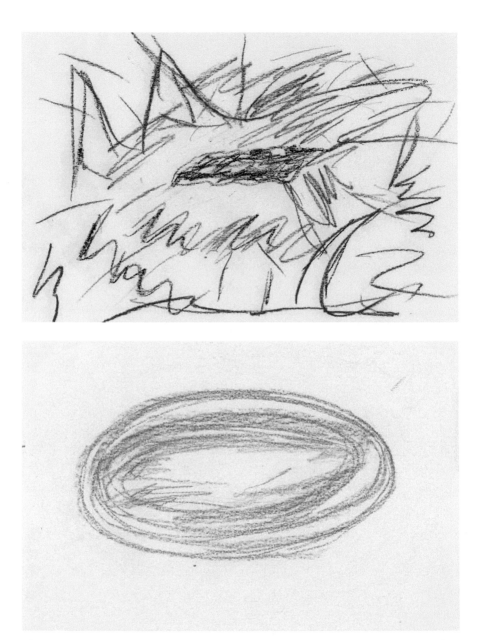

Figure 7. Two pictures created before and after fever therapy on the same day. The images were created spontaneously; the only stipulation was for the patient to express their mood intuitively and directly using colors. On the day after the fever therapy, our patients regularly report feeling relieved and revitalized, both physically and mentally.

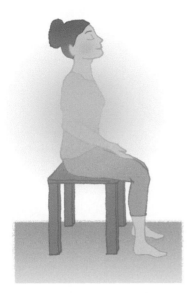

Figure 8. Affirmations work most powerfully when we focus on them, giving the words a special color or imagined light energy and combining them with a physical sensation.

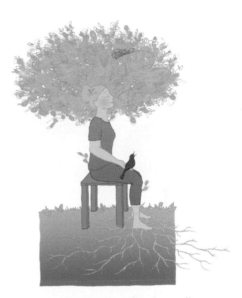

Figure 9. Healing meditations align consciousness and promote coherence.

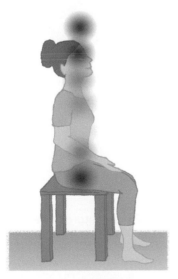

Figure 10. Healing Meditation 4: Meditating with the Seven Chakras

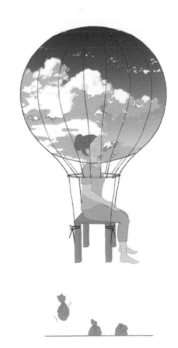

Figure 11. Healing Meditation 5: The Light Meditation

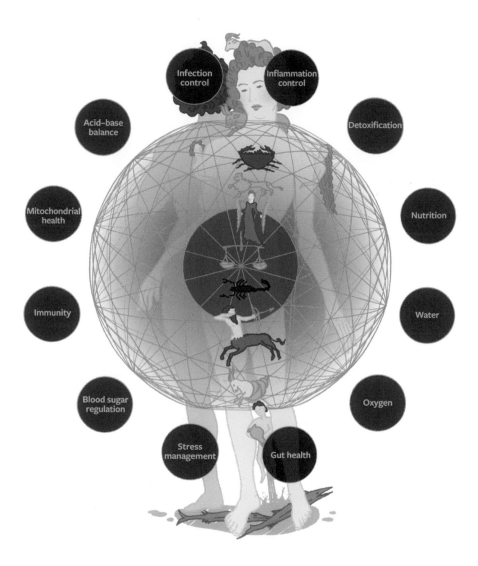

Figure 12. Cancer is a constant reminder of the equilibrium nature of health on which to build a fulfilling life.

stick to the amounts mentioned here so that the negative effects of alcohol consumption do not outweigh the positive properties of resveratrol. White wine contains only about a tenth of the amount of resveratrol compared to red wine and thus has no value for health. In addition to the health-promoting resveratrol, red wine, unlike white wine, also contains polyphenols, which include anthocyanins, with decidedly powerful antioxidant properties.

CREATINE

Half of creatine is ingested through food and half is produced by the body. It is essential for the functioning of the body and especially for the muscles, brain, and sensory organs. When food is preserved, however, it is broken down and is then no longer available to the body. Creatine can inhibit the growth of malignant tumor cells and simultaneously make them more sensitive to chemotherapy and radiotherapy.

Measures to Strengthen (and Increase) the Mitochondria

THERMOGENESIS

For most of us, an ice bath is probably out of the question for practical and conditional reasons, but with regular cold stimuli such as whole-body showers, temporary freezing or partial applications such as Kneipp water jets, treading water, and dew walking or something similar, we can promote the proliferation of mitochondria and stimulate respiration in the cells. Of course, the effect of exposure to cold over the whole body has a much greater effect on the organism than just partial stimuli. Even brown adipose tissue, which has a particularly large number of mitochondria but regresses during adolescence, can be reactivated. In addition, the immune system is strengthened in general.

ALTITUDE TRAINING

Although altitude training also increases and improves mitochondria and their function, it is certainly not feasible for most of us. Known to competitive athletes as a form of training and to tourists in very high mountain regions, the positive effects of hypoxia training can be achieved in the IHHT described above, which is even more intensive but can be carried out only with the appropriate technical equipment available in clinics.

ENDURANCE TRAINING

If the energy requirement increases during endurance training, new mitochondria must be formed. Interestingly, new mitochondria are formed not only in the muscle cells but also in the brain. The reason is perhaps the brain's high energy expenditure for motor control.

KETOGENIC DIET

The ketogenic diet has already been mentioned in section 3.2.10. By avoiding or greatly reducing carbohydrates, the body must rely on fat as an energy source. However, it should be discussed on an individual basis with a doctor how long and to what extent this dietary form of nutrition can be implemented. A strict ketogenic diet should not be followed permanently and should be selected—if at all—for an individual by an experienced doctor or therapist and supported accordingly.

INTERMITTENT FASTING

Intermittent fasting is also called interval fasting and does not describe a certain form of fasting, but a certain eating rhythm. In contrast to other forms of fasting, with intermittent fasting we eat normally, but at specific intervals. These intervals can be between twelve and sixteen hours, depending on how the organism in question can cope. If, for example, we eat our last meal at about six o'clock in the evening, by six o'clock the next morning our body will have already gone twelve hours without eating; with a late breakfast at ten o'clock, it will have already been sixteen hours.

Within these intervals, the body starts to produce ketone bodies (as in the ketogenic diet) from the available reserves for energy production.

This eating behavior relieves the organism, since our genetic heritage is to be able to manage without solid food for longer periods of time. The fact that we have an overabundance of—too rich—food or meals available to us at almost any time of day or night is a very modern development that is not adapted to our organism and our work or exercise behavior. Intermittent fasting improves, among other things, the mitochondria's ability to oxidize fatty acids and reduces oxidative stress. The insulin sensitivity of our cells is promoted and thus slows down cell aging. Individual fasting days can also relieve the organism and contribute to strengthening the mitochondria.

3.10 **The Acid–Base Balance**

3.10.1 **Living Between Acids and Bases**

Similar to the topic of healthy nutrition, we also find the assessment of the importance of the acid–base balance for our organism presented very differently in medical literature and practice. In naturopathy, the treatment of a disturbed acid–base balance (ABB) occupies an important place. The ABB is a differentiated interplay between different (more) alkaline and (more) acidic environments in the body, which can vary depending on the organ, tissue, or body region. In the stomach, for example, an acidic environment is needed to metabolize food. The skin's protective acid mantle is also, as the name suggests, an acidic environment that inhibits the growth of fungi and bacteria. In organs such as the pancreas and intestines, conditions are more alkaline, just like in the blood. The acidified food from the stomach, for example, is *moderated* in the pancreas by the secreted pancreatic juice and neutralized during the passage from the small intestine to the large intestine. The equilibrium of the ABB is disturbed daily by, for example, acid-forming food or too little exercise or oxygen, but normally every organism is able to maintain the different acidic, alkaline, or neutral environments in the body and to counteract hyperacidity by means of a sophisticated buffer system. If the body's buffer system can no longer cushion or neutralize excessive acid formation, the ABB is tipped, resulting in hyperacidity. A distinction is made between acute hyperacidity, also called acute acidosis, and chronic acidosis (from the Latin *acidum*).

In complementary medicine, an out-of-balance ABB is of decisive importance in the understanding of the occurrence of many diseases of civilization. Chronic acidosis is the milder, but more persistent form of hyperacidity. Although the acid load of the organism manifests itself in symptoms such as fatigue, lack of concentration, tiredness, susceptibility to infections, skin problems, digestive disorders, gastrointestinal problems, weight gain, and depression, these symptoms occur insidiously and gradually. Chronic acidosis can lead to further secondary diseases such as arthrosis, arthritis, rheumatism, and gout or can aggravate already existing diseases.

In orthodox medicine at university hospitals, the subject of ABB is dealt with almost exclusively in the intensive medical treatment of severe metabolic disorders such as acute kidney failure or severe respiratory disorders. This form is also called acute acidosis, is life-threatening (caused, for example, by poisoning with opiates or sleeping pills, by foreign bodies in the lungs, or due to kidney failure), and usually requires immediate intensive medical treatment.

Our interest, however, is directed toward the subtle acid–base shifts in our tissues, which are to do with the pH values going up and down, as well as the significant reaction of our immune system and our detoxification organs, which in turn influence the energy production of our mitochondria. But first, some basics will help to clarify what we are talking about here.

3.10.2 What Is an Acid and What Is a Base?

Everyone knows that an acid has a characteristic acidic taste. The sensation is a reaction of actively contracting. Bases, on the other hand, have a more oily-soapy, bitter effect on the sense of taste. For the biochemical effect on our metabolism, however, the taste impression can be very deceptive. Lemons are metabolized as alkaline in the body, and too much sugar, meat, and alcohol have an overacidifying effect, as already shown in section 3.2, "Healthy Nutrition and Health-Promoting Dietary Supplements Using the Example of the Twelve Vital Fields," page 36.

In order to get an answer to the question of the significance of the ABB for our health, we have to address the nature of biochemical reactions, namely in relation to the giving off or taking up of electrical charges, which take place everywhere in animate nature—in our body, throughout life, in a constant interplay of acidic and alkaline substances and their reactions. In the process, the smallest electrical charges or particles—called protons and electrons in physics—are pushed back and forth between the reaction partners. This is also called a redox reaction if it is an electron exchange, and an acid–base reaction if it is a proton, or hydrogen-ion, exchange.

In the chemical processes of reduction, these small particles and their electrical charges oscillate back and forth between electron donation (the reducing agent is oxidized in the process) and electron uptake (the reducing partner is reduced in the process). In the acid–base reaction, in comparable processes, it is the proton donation or proton uptake.

Redox reactions = back and forth oscillation of electrons

Acid–base reactions = back and forth oscillation of protons (positively
   charged hydrogen H+)

The pH value and the dynamics of the redox reactions form the biochemical basis for all metabolic processes in our body. This is reason enough for us to take a closer look at these metabolic processes, the ABB, in order to understand what promotes our health and what inhibits it.

First, a few basics: Hydrogen acts as a reducing agent in our body fluids, gives off electrons, and is itself oxidized to free hydrogen ions (H+). Oxygen (O_2) behaves in exactly the opposite way: It accepts electrons and is itself reduced. In Latin, oxygen is called *oxygenium*, "the oxidizing," and *oxyd* in Greek means "acidic."

The pH value of a solution, for example, of a certain body fluid, gives us the measure of the concentration of free hydrogen ions (H+), mathematically seen as a negative, decadic logarithm. Here, pH stands for *pondus hydrogenii* (Latin *pondus* meaning "weight" and *hydrogenium* meaning "hydrogen"), which essentially means "weight of hydrogen."

A pH value of 7 therefore means that the concentration of H+ is equal to 10^{-7}. The lower the pH value, the more hydrogen ions the solution contains and the more acidic the environment.

The higher the pH value, the more alkaline the solution is. A change in the pH value of 0.3 corresponds to a doubling or halving of the concentration of hydrogen ions. As explained above, our blood with a pH value of 7.45 at body temperature is in the slightly alkaline range. It is kept stable by various highly complex buffering processes under all circumstances and for as long as possible.

Our connective tissue, on the other hand, is in the neutral range (around 7.0) under normal conditions, and the pH value of a human cell is 6.9. At body temperature, this corresponds to the neutral point. The cell thus has about three times the concentration of hydrogen compared to the blood.

The pH value is also of crucial importance for the activity of enzymes in our cells and tissues. Various digestive enzymes, such as pepsin located in the stomach, work better in acidic environments, and others, such as trypsin that is active in the small intestine, work better in alkaline (i.e., basic) environments. If we look at these biochemical processes from a more over-view level, we can see the fundamental phenomenon of life processes in our body: the back-and-forth flow of energy. Life depends on the continuous bouncing back and forth of electrons, in other words, immaterial energy. In this way, we can also understand why both the rigidity of an energy flow in general and the rigidity of acid–base reactions in particular can be accom-panied by health problems and disease in our organism. For it is precisely this immobility in the ABB that occurs when the factors of the vital field described in this book remain out of balance. Chronic tissue overacidifica-tion is a paralysis of the system that needs to be treated therapeutically. It occurs with a prolonged unhealthy and one-sided diet, when we move too little, and for example, when we continuously breathe too shallowly due to stress. We come full circle here, too. The consequences of hyperacidity are the basis for further complaints.

The natural balancing of hyperacidity is the task of the basic matrix of our organism, that is, the network of highly polymeric sugar–protein complexes that, like a molecular sieve, enables and biochemically modulates the entire exchange of substances from the capillaries of our blood and lymphatic sys-tem to the cell and back again.

The negative charges of the matrix sugar surfaces of our cells, called gly-cocalyx, are of great importance for the ABB. They can absorb and neutralize excess protons as carriers of the acid effect. However, if the buffer capacity is exceeded (see above), there are far-reaching problems with cell regulation.

"Strictly speaking, the cell concept is only a morphological abstraction. Biologically, it cannot be used without the living environment of the cell." This is how the Viennese professor of histology and embryology Alfred Pischinger described the weakness of Rudolf Virchow's cellular pathology (see introduction), which wanted to define the concept of disease exclusively in terms of disorders within the individual cell. However, the cell and its behavior cannot be fully understood without the surrounding system of basic regulation. And it is precisely in this surrounding system that the con-stantly occurring redox reactions and shifts of the ABB take place.

Blood, which is everywhere in the organism, has, among other things, the task of keeping the pH value in the body stable and neutralizing overacidified areas. It contains various buffer substances that are supposed to carry out this balancing at any given time: phosphates, proteins such as hemoglobin or matrix proteins, and sodium hydrogen carbonate. The latter is coupled to respiration and can eliminate virtually unlimited amounts of volatile acids by releasing carbonic acid (CO_2), provided we breathe sufficiently deeply and effectively (see section 3.4, "Oxygen, Breathing, and Cancer Growth," page 82). If the buffering capacity of our blood is depleted by an acid-forming diet, lack of exercise, and stress, it can no longer perform its pH-balancing function. And this is exactly the point: Chronic hyperacidity goes hand in hand with a depleted and no longer functioning buffer function of our blood.

3.10.3 Live Blood Analysis in the Dark Field Microscope: Indicator for Balancing and Vitalizing Therapies

The live blood analysis in the dark field microscope at a one-hundred- to four-hundred-fold magnification gives a good insight into the basic substance (matrix) of our body, but at the same time shows a whole series of phenomena that the practiced doctor must distinguish between. The rouleaux formation phenomenon often observed here—the sticking together of red blood cells into chains resembling stacks of coins—or the occurrence of protein precipitations between the blood cells is interpreted, among other things, as an indication of tissue overacidification, which is often still associated with an insufficient electrical charge of the cell membranes. From my twenty years of experience with dark field microscopy of live blood, I can confirm that these phenomena—blood cells sticking together and protein precipitations between the blood cells—are part of the usual picture of cancer patients' blood. Gradually, the more balanced the acid–base balance of the whole organism and the stronger the electrical membrane charge of the cells, the more this condition diminishes or disappears.

The live blood analysis serves the naturopathic doctor as an instrument to assess the basic substance and its vital parameters in the course of the treatments. As valuable as this method is to me, I nevertheless advise against using it to make statements about the diagnosis of cancer or other diseases or a possible overacidification. It is a supplementary examination method and is not suitable for diagnosing infections or cancer.

3.10.4 **The Acid–Base Balance and Its Importance for Inflammation and Cancer**

All inflammatory reactions are associated with a slight metabolic acidosis, or a metabolically induced hyperacidity, and are usually accompanied by increased activity of the sympathetic nervous system. The longer this state of permanent inflammation and sympathicotonia (the balance is shifted in favor of the sympathetic nervous system) lasts, the more the energy production of the cells living in this state is reduced. The consequence of this imbalance is both the loss of energy in the cells (reduced ATP production in the mitochondria) and the loss of the high degree of development and specialization, as well as the adaptation of the cells to the conditions of the biochemical composition of the fluid space between the cells (*basic substance* or also extracellular matrix according to Pischinger). The cell is in a sense "de-differentiated" and goes through the developmental stages back to the undifferentiated embryo cell. This is also called malignancy (from Latin *malignitas*, meaning "malice"), which in medicine describes a process that characterizes a disease or a course of disease with progressive destruction that can possibly also lead to the death of the diseased person. This condition is bad for the organism as a whole and can become dangerous, because these cells have the tendency to multiply unchecked and spread into the organism, forming metastases, although or precisely because they cultivate a "loner existence" and behave *dissocially*.

It is known that tumor cells increasingly pump protons out of the cell and thus overacidify their environment. The inner milieu of the tumor cells becomes too alkaline, the outer milieu too acidic, and a pathological imbalance occurs.

However, this knowledge is also used therapeutically, for example, in the treatment of stomach cancer with the help of proton pump inhibitors, which are supposed to prevent this increased proton output. If this overacidification is blocked or neutralized, immune cells can again reach the tumor cell unhindered and attack it. It is therefore of great importance not only for the state of health in general, but also for cancer in particular, to keep the ABB balanced or, if necessary, to bring it into balance so that the immune system can develop its greatest possible scope of action.

3.10.5 Overacidification and Measurement Methods

If you inform yourself about the topic of the balance of acids and bases, the pH-value measurements of saliva or urine are often still erroneously presented or recommended as meaningful. However, measurements of saliva and urine unfortunately say nothing about the pH ratios of our tissues, but rather allow conclusions to be drawn about what we have eaten in the last few hours and how we have got rid of acids and bases through excretion. I therefore advise my patients not to measure the pH value of urine or saliva themselves.

Measuring the pH of the blood does not help to determine the pH of the tumor and the peritumoral environment either, because the blood pH of our organism—as already mentioned—is kept constant under all circumstances. Certain substances of this buffer system can neutralize both acids and bases to a certain extent. However, if the blood pH changes, the person is seriously ill and needs intensive clinical treatment.

The only useful measurement of the blood to inform us about the tissue pH is the titration of blood using hydrochloric acid. This process is described in detail by Johan van Limburg Stirum in his book *Modern Acid-Base Medicine*. In simple terms, it measures how many drops (or microliters) of hydrochloric acid the blood can buffer before the buffering capacity fails and the pH value suddenly tips. The measurement result allows conclusions to be drawn about the ABB of the entire organism, but the process is complex and can be carried out only in practice with a great deal of time and only immediately after blood has been taken and with special equipment. Since the measurement must be taken immediately after the blood is taken, the blood cannot be sent to a laboratory to be measured.

It is known from basic research that cancer tumors produce high amounts of lactic acid (lactate) and that this leads to a local overacidification of the peritumoral environment around the tumor. This is one of the reasons why certain tumors can be attacked only with difficulty or not at all by the immune system: They successfully shield themselves in this way from the immune system, as it can hardly have an antitumor effect in overacidified areas.

It would be desirable to be able to directly measure tissue overacidification and its severity, since—as described at the beginning of this section—the consequences of overacidification can promote a further deterioration of the environment and stronger tumor growth or further secondary diseases. However, this is unfortunately not, or hardly, feasible in the practical everyday situation, because equipment would be needed for the tests described above, which is available only in research laboratories. Our recommendations regarding therapeutic measures for deacidification or detoxification of tissues and organs are therefore based on the knowledge obtained from basic research. We assume that cancer patients, as well as, for example, overweight patients or patients with a metabolic syndrome or autoimmune inflammations, have a more or less pronounced local tissue hyperacidity, depending on the stage of the disease, which we can effectively counteract with naturopathic measures.

3.10.6 The Complementary Deacidification Therapies

Diet

As a general recommendation, it would do many of us good to follow a more alkaline diet. Today's often hectic lifestyle; the choice of foods with an overabundance of animal fats, carbohydrates, and sugar; and the mass of processed foods lead to an imbalance of the ABB. One-sided diets produce more acidic metabolic products, and many one-sided diets also promote the overacidification of the organism. Fast food, convenience products, baked goods, and other "prepared" and packaged products contain artificial additives that do not belong in a healthy, vitalizing diet. It is therefore advisable to frequently take the time that is due not only for the meals themselves, but also for the purchase and preparation of food. As a special recommendation, we advise against people treating themselves on the basis of a pH value determination of the urine or saliva, by trying out or maintaining extreme diets, but instead, if a pronounced acid–base imbalance is suspected, to seek advice and guidance from experienced doctors or naturopaths.

The nutritional recommendations described in section 3.2, "Healthy Nutrition and Health-Promoting Dietary Supplements Using the Example of the Twelve Vital Fields," page 36, describe in their diversity, balance, freshness, and naturalness precisely those characteristics of healthy nutrition that also support and promote a balanced acid–base balance in an optimal way.

Basically, what was already recommended in the nutrition section also applies to a healthy, acid–base balancing diet. The basis here should also be a lot of fruits and vegetables, herbs, nuts, sprouts, and seeds, and these should make up the largest part of the daily diet. They are alkaline-promoting and rich in fiber, nutrients, and minerals that promote optimal metabolic function and support the buffer systems of the blood and organs. The proportion of carbohydrates should be lower and preferably consist of the whole grain or pseudo grain varieties already described. Meat, proteins, and fats should also be consumed less frequently, and good quality should be ensured. Animal products in particular, from meat and sausages to dairy products such as cow's milk, cheese, yogurt, quark, and cream—in that order—to eggs and animal fats should and probably can be reduced significantly in most cases. Sugar is also a strong acidifier and is still eaten every day by many people in excessive quantities.

Just as with any other form of nutrition, an acid–base balancing diet should also include an adequate intake of fluids such as water and unsweetened herbal teas. The fear that carbonated mineral water has a harmful effect on the ABB is unfounded. Only an insignificantly small proportion—less than 1 percent—of this compound of gas and water actually forms carbonic acid (H_2CO_3), which also remains stable for only fractions of a second. This means that sparkling water does not contribute to overacidification of the body. A healthy diet and a balanced ABB include the restriction of alcohol and nicotine alongside increased vegetable consumption.

The already mentioned increased breathing and the associated oxygen supply as well as a massage of the organs also have a balancing effect on the ABB. In addition to sports activities and physical exercise, it also helps to breathe consciously and deeply, not to stress or allow yourself to be stressed, and to establish abdominal breathing. Although we would like to encourage and call for exercise and sports, not everyone has to become a sports champion overnight, regardless of their physical or mental capabilities: Cycling more often, walking, or taking the stairs instead of the elevator are examples of advice that is given again and again but cannot be disregarded and can be incorporated into everyday life.

Depending on your fitness level, even regular walking—or, if possible, light jogging, raising the heart rate to no more than 120 beats per minute—is very beneficial.

Cardio training as a variation of endurance training can also be done at home or in the gym with the help of special equipment in order to support the ABB, among other things by improving the oxygen–carbon dioxide exchange and by sweating out acidic metabolic products. The function of the heart–lung system is also improved. If the organism is overtaxed, weakened by illness, or even emaciated, it makes sense to formulate small but feasible partial goals that can truly be achieved.

––––––––––

Via nutrition, breathing, and exercise, we come to the fourth area of the acid–base balancing, namely the inner approach or orientation. This, too, has already been mentioned or discussed in some places in this book, but it should be mentioned here again as a special module, as it is inseparably linked to the topics of health, well-being, and recovery. Our inner attitude or orientation in relation to the world is expressed not only in what we do and what we consume, but also in how we treat ourselves and others, how we evaluate ourselves and others, and how we feel as a result. Often, we feel that we come up against inner or outer boundaries, that we are restricted by certain circumstances or people, or that we are treated in a certain negative way. However, we can also reverse this direction through our inner attitude or inner orientation. With the practices presented in chapter 6, such as the healing meditations, inner life training exercises, mindfulness training, yoga, and other spiritual or mental methods that increase our well-being and reduce our stress, we can rebalance and reorient ourselves. This, in turn, will affect breathing, stress reduction, state of mind, well-being, and so forth, since metabolic processes can change and adapt, and new feelings, thoughts, and eventually actions can mature. In this sense, even the inner attitude is conducive to a balanced ABB, as we invariably do ourselves good with mindfulness and a conscious lifestyle.

In addition, we offer our patients the following therapy methods to balance or optimize the ABB.

Kneipp Applications and Water

In order to optimize blood circulation and oxygen supply in the entire organism, the tissues, and the organs, we prescribe Kneipp applications, consisting of alternating hot and cold water jets or showers on certain parts of the body. They not only stimulate blood circulation and thus detoxification, but also strengthen the mitochondrial function and the oxygen supply of the cells and have an acid–base balancing effect. The vast majority of Kneipp applications can also be carried out alone at home. If you have a garden or live near a body of water, you could start the day with water or dew treading to stimulate the organism and get rid of toxins such as excess acids. Drinking enough pure, filtered, or swirled water is one of the top commandments to support the ABB. The well-known priest and naturopath Sebastian Kneipp (1821–1897) therefore advocated the rule of thumb of drinking one glass of water per hour to provide the organism with sufficient fluid.

Alkaline baths (for example, as a full bath at home with an addition of alkaline minerals, such as sodium hydrogen carbonate) are also supportive for a balanced ABB, beneficial for the skin, and generally stimulate and balance the metabolism.

In chapter 6, we introduce you to further therapeutic measures for the regulation of the ABB, such as PEMF therapy, oxygen and ozone therapy, as well as exercise and sports, alkaline infusions, and specific food supplements that have an effect on the ABB.

3.11 Healing and Preventing Infections

3.11.1 Infection and Inflammation

If we compare our body to a house or inn, it reacts to uninvited "guests" with inflammation in order to "drive them out of the house." Examples of disease-causing invaders are bacteria, fungi, viruses, pathogenic molecules, prions, as well as singe-cell or multicell parasites. Infection is therefore defined as the invasion of disease-causing microorganisms and the settlement and multiplication of these small organisms in a host organism, in our case humans. In the process, the infecting organisms use the host's structures and processes, usually at the host's expense.

The Latin *inficere* means "to infect" or literally "to put into," while *immunis* means to be "free of" something. So the effort is always to eliminate, inactivate, or at least control what has entered, the trigger. The balance of power between the host (human being) and guest (infectious microorganism) determines the further course of the encounter. With a strong host, the multiplication of the "guests" is kept within a framework compatible with health.

The immune system is an interplay of different organs, cell types, and proteins, and the reaction of the immune system is a highly complex sequence of biochemical processes. With the aim of eliminating the cause or triggers, inflammation is therefore initially a natural and effective defense reaction of the body and thus an important component of the immune system and defense, and is biologically extremely useful in eliminating specific triggers.

Described in more detail, inflammation is a genetically determined program, which has been developed over millions of years, for repair and self-healing of damaged tissues in higher mammals, including humans.

We know it very well from everyday life. As soon as a foreign body enters our organism and damages tissue—be it a small splinter of wood that gets under the skin, physical forces in the form of hot water that we scald ourselves with, or a blow to the finger—this self-healing program begins: Within seconds, the organism starts doing everything to repair this injury quickly and effectively. First, with the help of the nervous system, pain signals tell us that the affected part of the body must be protected; then, the damaged tissue swells. This is an attempt to dilute the toxins that have accumulated there as a result of the damage, for example, from bursting cells, from immigrated dirt particles or microorganisms, and to flush them out through increased circulation of blood and lymph. At the same time, however, the building materials are brought in for repair. This generates hyperthermia and redness, and the original function is temporarily impaired.

With this, we have described the five classic symptoms of acute inflammation:

1. redness (Lat. *rubor*)
2. swelling (Lat. *tumor*)
3. overheating up to fever (Lat. *calor*)
4. pain (Lat. *dolor*)
5. functional limitation (Lat. function *laesa*)

———

All of this is aimed at transporting the correct biological building blocks through increased blood flow and plasma egress, as well as platelets and immune cells into the tissue through the dilated blood vessels to the site of the event or damage, so that the damaged and partially or completely perished cells can be replaced by new ones—sometimes also by scar tissue. The state of acute inflammation usually lasts a few days or a few weeks and should then subside again through sound self-regulation.

Sometimes, however, this does not succeed, inflammation is maintained, and an autoimmune disease develops. Section 3.12, "Chronic Inflammation: Silent Inflammation," page 150, deals with these circumstances.

Many of the inflammatory diseases can already be recognized by the terminological ending -*itis*, for example, the rheumatic inflammation arthritis, *Hashimoto's thyroiditis* (inflammation of the thyroid gland), the autoimmune intestinal inflammation *colitis ulcerosa* or Crohn's diseases, *gastritis*, *sinusitis*, *bronchitis*, chronic skin eczema, and others. It seems as if the organism has missed the right time to stop the inflammation and let it rest again. Overactivity with continued inflammation takes the place of a healthy willingness to react inflammatorily when necessary.

An infection can proceed in very different ways.

Peracute: rapid and dangerous, as the subsequent course of the disease is severe, often fatal

Acute: sudden onset, severe effects

Sub-acute: less severe, gradual, few symptoms, sometimes no noticeable symptoms at all

Chronic: gradual onset, prolonged, lasting longer than three months according to the current medical definition

Relapsing: recurring with the same trigger or pathogen

Latent: smoldering secretly, asymptomatic, lasting a long time with intervening clinically silent phases

---

According to the latest calculations, infections play a major role in the development of the later condition in about 15 percent of all cancers. This is significantly more than the proportion of the cancer risk inherited through genes, which is estimated to be only about 5 percent.

The infectious diseases that significantly increase the risk of cancer include, above all:

Helicobacter pylori, the stomach bacterium that a quarter of the German population carries. The bacterium is responsible for about 75 percent of all stomach ulcers. Such chronic inflammations of the stomach mucosa, which are perpetuated by an infection, can particularly often develop into stomach cancer.

The two hepatitis viruses B and C are the most important risk factors for the development of liver cancer. About 8,500 people in Germany develop liver cancer every year. Since 2003 the number of patients diagnosed with liver cancer in the United States has more than doubled, from 16,000 to 35,000 new cases per year.

HPV, the human papilloma virus, is causally linked to cervical cancer. The much rarer cancers such as penis and anal cancer are also associated with HPV infections.

―――――――

Another field that has not been studied much by scientific medical research is that of intracellular infections. It is known that a whole range of microorganisms can multiply inside human cells, including *Borrelia* and *Chlamydia*, for example.

A group of microbiologists at the University of Würzburg in Germany is currently investigating the connection between chlamydial infections and ovarian cancer, and evidence is accumulating that a chlamydial infection may be linked to the development of ovarian cancer. According to the Würzburg scientists, chlamydiae activate certain signals that promote their survival and protect them from apoptotic (pre-programmed) cell death. This leads to the degeneration into a cancerous behavior of the cells and ultimately to cancer.

―――――――

In 1882, the medical doctor and founder of bacteriology Robert Koch (1843–1910) was the first to find tuberculosis bacteria in the blood of people suffering from tuberculosis. The invading tubercle bacteria (*Mycobacterium tuberculosis*) were believed to be the only cause of this disease and it was believed that the blood of healthy people was free of bacteria, or sterile. Today, this supposition is considered outdated.

Louis Pasteur (1822–1895), the French chemist, physicist, biochemist and cofounder of medical microbiology, recognized at the end of his seventy-two-year life: "Le Mikrobe n'est rien. Le Terrain est tout" (*The microbe is nothing. The terrain—the environment—is everything*). With this conviction, Pasteur already referred to the vital field, aspects of which we are dealing with here. Important modern microbiologists such as the American professor Lida H. Mattman, PhD (1912–2008), or Gitte Jensen, founder of NIS Labs in Oregon, have gained a different understanding of the relationship between bacteria and host organism and replaced the term *infection* with *microbe–host relationship* (Jensen), since virtually all mammals, including humans, are always *infected*, or constantly inhabited by microorganisms, and only sometimes pathologically afflicted. Who or what decides on the course and outcome of an infection, on being affected by microorganisms?

Again, the conclusion is that it is not a single factor, but an interplay of several factors, which I call in their totality the *vital field*.

3.11.2 Increasing Coherence as a Therapeutic Concept for Infections

By vitalizing and optimizing the interplay of the various processes or subfactors of the vital field, chronic infections will either heal better or retreat to latent, nonactive forms, and thus no longer disturb healthy life. Sometimes it is necessary to kill the infectious microorganism. This can be done either with synthetic drugs such as modern antibiotics or with natural anti-infective substances such as *Artemisia annua* (wormwood), oregano oil, mustard oils, and many others.

However, without a rehabilitation of the whole organism, such anti-infective therapy will always run the risk of suppressing the infection for only a certain time until it returns because of the weakened host. Therefore, with all antibiotic therapies, probiotic therapies are of utmost importance, either afterward or in parallel to antibiosis (treatment with antibiotics, such as penicillin and others).

Against the background of the vital field hypothesis presented here, the problem of infection as a disease seems to be very similar to that of cancer, and a direct connection between both types of disease, which are linked by inflammation, is obvious. However, for both forms of disease, this also means that there is no such thing as a sterile, or noninfected, human organism, just as there is no such thing as a human being free of cancer cells. Not every infection leads to a disease with symptoms, and the presence of a few thousand cancer cells in humans seems to be the natural state of the organism. But when does an infection and when does living together with cancer cells become a disease? Whenever the sum of the disturbances of the vital field has exceeded a sufficiently pathological threshold, and the coherent homeostasis, or the interrelated self-regulation and the complex occurrence of health, can no longer be maintained.

In the sense of the holistic approach in this book, I recommend that you look for stimuli on all twelve levels of the vital field, in order to be able to effectively transition infections—acute as well as chronic—into health.

3.12 Chronic Inflammation: Silent Inflammation

Inflammation occurs in our body everywhere that is exposed to a nonphysiological stimulus, one that does not correspond to normal life processes and exceeds a healthy degree. Such a stimulus can be caused by various influences: by the penetration of bacteria, viruses, fungi; by the influence of chemical substances such as acids or metabolic hyperacidity (for example, in gout); by physical changes such as heat and cold; by mechanical forces such as in the case of a bruise or strain; or by aggressive electromagnetic waves such as UV light (sunburn) or ionizing/radioactive radiation (radiotherapy).

In the previous section, acute inflammation was presented as a consequence and *protective* or *repair measure* of an infection. As already mentioned in this context, the organism sometimes does not succeed in completely shutting down the inflammatory reaction again, and a smoldering low-level inflammation remains, which one does not even notice or hardly notices. The smoldering or silent inflammation is the younger sister of acute inflammation. This silent inflammation is also called chronic smoldering inflammation and is the engine of all chronic diseases in modern man. In most cases, it also plays a key role in cancer.

Chronic Smoldering or "Silent" Inflammation

An infection usually leads to an inflammatory reaction of the organism. In this way, we can consider chronic infection as a cause of chronic inflammation. One of the important and central factors in the development of cancer is precisely this chronic inflammation, which very often goes unnoticed, and therefore is considered to be silent or smoldering. The attempt at self-healing through inflammation gets stuck in a behavioral pattern without being able to overcome and eliminate the triggering cause.

Even if we do not or no longer notice the chronic or low-level inflammation—because it does not hurt, we do not develop a fever to overcome it, and the swelling and functional restriction are thus below the perceptual threshold—it nevertheless decisively changes the basic biochemical factors for cellular life in this part of the tissue if it persists in this smoldering state of inflammation. Acidification and oxygen depletion due to the formation of too many free oxygen radicals—which have a cell-damaging effect in excess—or an immunological misdirection and change in the energy metabolism of the cells are the result. This smoldering inflammation is one of the most common but also one of the most dangerous breeding grounds for the development of cancer cells, because if it is not eliminated in time, it grows into a cancerous disease.

The latency period from the beginning of uncontrolled cancer cell growth to the emergence of a palpable and visible cancer node is estimated to be several years. Transferring a chronic inflammation into a temporary, therapeutically triggered acute inflammation is one of the modes of action of treatment by whole-body hyperthermia. By artificially triggering a fever, the low-level inflammation that has become chronic can often be transferred into a normal, healthy state by transforming it into an acute inflammation (for more on this, see chapter 6). The therapeutic concept of hormesis plays a decisive role here: *Hormesis* (Greek, "stimulation" or "impetus" meaning *adaptive response*) is a term used by Paracelsus to describe that small doses of harmful or toxic substances can have a positive effect on organisms by triggering a useful healing response. Today, it is defined more broadly and describes the principle of providing the body with a therapeutic stimulus through which it regains its ability to self-regulate. We will discuss this principle in more detail on the subject of oxygen therapies and heat therapy (hyperthermia).

The development of cancer and cancerous behavior of cells in a tissue or organ can be described as *degenerate* inflammation. Cancer is in many cases a malignant variant of inflammation. For this reason, many anticancer agents are also and above all anti-inflammatory agents.

Turmeric, resveratrol, digestive enzymes, omega-3 fats, acetylsalicylic acid, or even the synthetic anti-inflammatory drug celecoxib are successful in the treatment of cancer because they inhibit the inflammatory reactions.

Nf-Kappa-B is an important regulatory and key factor in this process, which, as a biochemical regulatory protein, switches certain genes on and off, that is, DNA sections that function like biochemical programs. These cellular programs in the genetic material of our cell nuclei can regulate our highly complex immune system between inflammation or cellular cancer defense. If this genetic "switch" is set to "inflammation," then certain immunological defense mechanisms that are able to recognize and eat up cancer cells can no longer work sufficiently well. Cancer cells are then no longer recognized by the immune system and grow uninhibited into a lump that, once it reaches a certain size, sends metastases into the surrounding area via blood and lymph.

Cancer is a potentially fatal disease primarily for this reason, because it migrates through metastases into the organism and very often into vital organs, penetrates these more and more, and, if no successful therapy stops this, destroys the entire organism. Preventing metastasis and interrupting the vicious circle of inflammation, immunological cancer attack, and thus unhindered cancer growth is therefore one of the most important tasks of cancer therapy. Natural inhibitors of Nf-Kappa-B, the important transcription factor for immune regulation, are, for example, allicin from the common onion, genistein from soy, quercetin from fruit peels, curcumin from turmeric (this is the spice plant *Curcuma longa*, which gives curry its yellow color), gingko, epigallocatechin gallate from green tea, and tocotrienols (substances similar to vitamin E), which are found in red palm oil and black cumin oil, among other things.

Extracts of oregano, coffee, thyme, clove, and walnut have been shown to significantly reduce excessive Nf-kappa-B levels in both laboratory tests (in vitro) and animal tests (in vivo). In this context, naturopathy also speaks of "inflammatory foci." These can be: chronically inflamed throat and tonsils, chronically inflamed glands such as the ovaries or the prostate, chronically inflamed tooth roots (especially after root fillings), or chronically inflamed mucous membranes in the gastrointestinal tract. The restoration of these foci is therefore of particular importance. A single focal point can noticeably worsen the highly sensitive immunological balance between inflammatory activity and cancer defense.

As a practical consequence, some examinations should therefore be carried out. These include, for example, the examination of inflammation parameters such as C-reactive protein (CRP), ferritin, blood cell sedimentation rate (BSR), and others in the blood. CRP is a protein body that is formed in the liver and released into the blood. This protein belongs to the acute phase proteins whose concentration increases in the blood during inflammatory diseases. In the same way, the ferritin value (Lat. *ferrum* meaning "iron") should also be examined, which can be increased by the acute phase reaction in the context of inflammatory processes. With a test for BSR, it can be determined how quickly the red blood cells of a blood sample are sedimented within an hour in a special tube. This value can serve as an indication of inflammation in the body.

The intestinal flora and intestinal immunology (the immune system and defense mechanisms of the intestine) should also be examined and, if necessary, remedied with appropriate orthomolecular substances (vitamins, minerals, micronutrients) and pre- and probiotics. For lasting intestinal health and relief in terms of a resistant microbiome, the diet should be changed.

The mouth and jaw area may be examined with a panoramic X-ray to assess root-filled teeth and, if necessary, possible inflammation foci are subsequently remedied. But also all other possible sources of inflammation in the body (these include, for example, tonsils, sinuses, skin and nails, and glands) should be localized and cured. As stated in section 3.2.1, "The Anti-Inflammatory Diet," page 39, pro-inflammatory influences (for example, hyperacidity, sugar, pork, hydrogenated fats, or synthetic substances in the diet) should be avoided and the intake of anti-inflammatory substances (for example, digestive enzymes, omega-3 fats, fiber, cruciferous vegetables, citrus fruits, turmeric, or coconut fat) should be intensified. The diet should be changed to a general anti-inflammatory diet. Section 3.2.1 therefore highlights essential points and compiles important information.

Chapter Four

Balance: Everything in Flux

Panta rhci!
—HERACLITUS

Everything flows! These words, attributed to the Greek philosopher Heraclitus (around 520 to 460 BC), so succinctly express what is a basic phenomenon of all living things: the flowing equilibrium. Biologists call it homeostasis.

Every moment of our lives, our metabolism is subject to a constant buildup and breakdown, which dissolves the structures of our cells and organs, only to rebuild and reassemble them in a meaningful and orderly manner in the next moment, before they disintegrate again. Although we perceive life as a constant state, this up and down, this coming into being and passing away, is the basic principle of our world. Our body, with the help of which we physically express our personality, also follows this principle through an active metabolism. Only the lens in our eye and the enamel of our teeth are exempt from this constant building up and breaking down of our life. This constant coming into being and passing away of organic structures affects not only our bodies but also the smallest parts, the subatomic particles or waves. Everything visible in the universe is made up of these particles. Quantum physicists teach us: Matter and the particles that it is made up of disappear and come into being in a constant interplay that takes place at the speed of light. Matter is therefore only apparently stationary and is more like a "standing wave" than something rigid.

In a workshop I attended, Bruce Lipton (American biologist, professor and cofounder of epigenetics) described the essence of the atoms that make up matter not as solid "building blocks" but as tiny "tornadoes" that rotate around their axis at the speed of light. The matter that appears to us as solid is based on the vortex of energy rotating at unimaginably fast speeds. From the outside, mind, will, and matter appear to be separate from each other.

But matter is—to a certain extent and under certain circumstances—open to change: Forces from our consciousness act on forces in our body. Consciousness acts on moving energy, and perhaps this is the reason why we can actively and effectively intervene in our organism with our will, or our directed consciousness. With this understanding, we can also approach, for example, the everyday *miracle* that our will intervenes in our body every time we send a movement impulse via our brain into our limbs with the help of our consciousness.

Can we also pass on such impulses to our immune system? Psycho-immunology undoubtedly answers this question with a "yes" (see section 6.1.7, "Stress Reduction," page 191). We just have to find the right language that our organism understands. Feelings seem to reach our organism much more strongly than mere thoughts. While a *cool* thought hardly influences our organism, positive feelings of joy, security, or enthusiasm, as well as negative feelings of fear, guilt, or shame can have a direct and even measurable effect—as recent studies have shown—on the production of messenger substances and hormones in our organism. We will come back to this in section 6.2, "How to Practice Inner Life Training," page 205.

If some of the twelve vital fields described in chapter 3 are permanently out of balance, these out-of-balance fields can endanger our health or, in the worst case, develop carcinogenic effects. If the ability to swing back and forth, to swing back into a phase of balance is lost, the flow of life comes to a standstill and something—the toxin, the deficiency, the surplus, too much or too little or the absence of springing back into the lightness of life—gets in the way of the self-balancing swinging of all living things.

The German philosopher and poet Friedrich Schiller (1759–1805) described this lightness of life in his notes (in letter form), "On the Aesthetic Education of Man." This lightness leads man again and again to the *center* and thus to freedom by swinging from one pole of the "oppressive barbarian" to the other pole of the helplessly "vulnerable savage." If this movement is miss-ing—described in Schiller's work as "play drive" and "lightness"—we remain in an unhealthy state or extreme.

Those who keep the twelve vital fields in flow, so that the state of balance can also be set again and again, will thereby not only counteract the danger of contracting cancer, but will also be able to observe a strengthening of their whole life (see figure 4 in the color insert).

In my experience with the vital field, being vital in this comprehensive sense also makes us more open to fantasy, creativity, and our life dream, the realization of which is our deepest life motive and our inner life force.

The dissonance of an illness and the resulting pain can and should be a sign for us, with the help of which we become aware of something that has temporarily or perhaps already for a long time escaped our attention because something else always seemed to be more important.

Therefore, a conscious and sustainable recovery process includes recognizing or becoming aware (again) of one's life motive. Dr. Kelly Turner—American researcher, lecturer, and consultant in the field of inte-grative cancer research—came across this connection in her research and describes it as one of nine crucial grounds to be able to cure cancer. In her empirical work, *Radical Remission: Surviving Cancer Against All Odds*, she pres-ents these nine healing factors, and she names "profound reasons for life," which people who have overcome cancer told her about, as essential.

Personally, therefore, it seems to be true that health is never fixed, but always in flux. "When will I finally be healthy?" or "Will I ever be completely healthy again?" are questions that my patients often ask me. My answer is always that healthy is something that we always "become" and has to be gained every day. As children, we are not yet aware of this. As adults, however, we can become aware of it so that we can face the oscillating balance of our lives in such a way that we can do the right thing, initiate the right countermovement and the right behavior when an illness has put us in an unbalanced position.

One and All
To make anew creation
So it doesn't shield itself to death
Is the eternal vital task.

What has not been, now it will manifest
To become the purest sun and colorful earth.
No way it must stand still.
It's supposed to move on, to act creatively
To morph and change,
It only seems to stand still for a moment,
The eternal moves in all that is:
To nothingness it has to fall,
In order to prevail as being.[7]

—JOHANN WOLFGANG VON GOETHE (1749–1832)

———————

We will now take a look at the many ways in which we can improve our health or help our body to regain its balance when it shows symptoms of illness or even seems to be stuck in illness.

Chapter Five

Complementary Oncology

5.1 Creating Synergies: A Key Objective of Integrative Medicine

In the world of conventional medicine, naturopathic or complementary integrative medicine is often viewed as a separate field one might resort to when there are no longer any conventional treatments left that follow the guidelines and patients have "nothing left to lose." The term *guidelines* refers to a set of treatment guidelines that are recommended to patients as standard. The guidelines put forward treatment strategies (e.g., surgery, chemotherapy, antihormonal therapy, radiation, antibody therapy) for which scientific studies are available, and they outline what the studies say about the effects, advantages, and disadvantages of these individual therapies on patients.

But biological, holistic medicine takes a completely different perspective. It considers conventional medicine to be a specialist medical field, for which large, generally recognized studies are available. A lot of the recommendations presented in this book, such as healthy eating, detoxification, and stress reduction, constitute the essential groundwork for any medical treatment in the self-conception of naturopathy. Beyond that, these elements are considered steps that should be taken as a matter of course for a health-conscious, disease-preventive life. Integrative medicine is the combined practice of nutritional medicine, biological medicine (e.g., detoxification and the use of vitamins and minerals in effective doses), therapeutic use of relaxation techniques, and conventional medicine. Integrative medicine is constantly seeking synergies—interactions between substances, forces, and living beings that mutually foster one another—that constitute the best, most effective, and most harmonious course of therapy for the individual. *Harmonious* treatment, in the complementary integrative medicine sense, means establishing a personalized course of treatment for the individual, which takes into account mind, body, and spirit.

What is uniformly considered, treated as, or declared "advantageous" in an evaluation of a large study with many participants is not necessarily the right thing for every person. In these kinds of conditions in particular, it is often impossible to take into account or investigate quality of life and the individual circumstances of those affected.

Individualized medicine highlights the absurdity of studying all important aspects of treatment—all issues related to the disease and factors involved in the healing possibilities—exclusively in large scientific studies carried out in advance. Even the largest and most costly form of modern research study—the double-blind randomized study, which sometimes includes a placebo control group and generally divides several hundred patients into different study groups at random—is not immune to errors or misinterpretations. In placebo-controlled trials, one group of volunteers is given the active ingredient or new drug to be investigated, and the other group is given a placebo, a drug without any active ingredients. When evaluating these studies, however, important individual factors such as diet, intake of dietary supplements, or natural remedies, as well as certain mental, psychological, and genetic dispositions, are not usually taken into account. As such, the fact that the results of any such study are considered to have an absolute informative value should be questioned. Results should not be considered the "only truth" or without alternative.

I am therefore not surprised when new, subsequent studies are carried out that come to the opposite conclusions or strongly question certain conclusions drawn from the original study.

Another common misconception is the idea that anything that has not been proven effective by large studies of this kind is, by definition, ineffective. The fact, for example, that no double-blind studies have been carried out on the effectiveness of using a hot water bottle to treat abdominal pain does not ultimately prove that doing so does not have a positive (anticonvulsant) effect. The effect simply hasn't been "proven" in any study thus far.

This book acknowledges the highly complex nature of human biology, both in the context of cancer and in general, and therefore takes a poly-pragmatic point of view. In other words, we assume that in the case of cancer, a healthy diet is more beneficial than poor nutrition, that good liver detoxification is better than poor, that mental well-being is better than constant stress, and so forth, regardless of the fact that a large scientific study does not exist for each of these factors. Despite billions invested into research, cancer does not seem to be curable in over 50 percent of cases. We therefore recommend polypragmatic, individualized treatment methods to all of our patients.

5.1.1 Are Naturopathic Complementary Medical Treatments and Companion Therapies Dangerous?

Time and again, people express the opinion that complementary medical treatments could weaken the effects of "real" treatments, conventional medical treatments, and are therefore dangerous. Since hardly any studies have been carried out on the subject of interactions between naturopathic and conventional medical treatments, we as doctors have to rely on our general technical understanding and experience. In my thirty years working as a doctor and having read specialist literature since my time as a student, I have not come across a study that describes or evaluates the therapies presented in this book as dangerous. Patients undergoing chemotherapy or radiation therapy can benefit from eating healthily and being mindful about the detoxification of their organs, especially during these strenuous treatments. Any exceptions must always be considered and discussed on an individual basis. Generally speaking, however, these recommendations apply.

Naturopathic treatments can, of course, also have side effects. It is known, for example, that the anticancer agent artemisinin, which comes from Chinese mugwort, can lead to a reduction in the number of red blood cells if used in (too) high doses. However, an experienced doctor will take this into account and ensure they treat their patients in a safe manner.

Chapter 6 deals with the most common side effects of complementary therapies and drugs.

5.1.2 What Are Some of the Warnings That Should Be Taken into Consideration?

There are a few things I'd like to warn my readers about, especially in regard to cancer and other diseases that can seem hopeless. There are certain factors to take into account, often related to an urgent desire for healing on the part of the patient on the one hand, and a frequent lack of a holistic understanding on the part of the practitioner on the other.

Anyone looking on the internet today for alternative cancer treatments, for example, will unfortunately find not only serious information, but also a lot of dubious, often fraudulent information. Among those providing information are dangerous charlatans, who make outrageous claims and emphasize certain half-truths that become untenable promises of salvation.

One example of this is the series of claims made by an Italian doctor who lost his medical license years ago but continued to illegally treat patients regardless, using alkaline infusions. He publicly advertised his work using this statement: "Cancer is a fungus and is cured by injecting basic agents such as sodium bicarbonate." Nothing about this statement is true!

By contrast, it has been truthfully established that certain tumors can sometimes be colonized by fungi and other microorganisms. Antimicrobial treatment and alkalizing measures can be useful in such cases, as they positively influence the environment by stabilizing or balancing it. They do not, however, guarantee spontaneous healing.

There are also claims circulating that vitamin C and B_{17}, better known by its chemical name, amygdalin, cure cancer. These claims are also completely false! It would be correct to state that in many cases, high doses of vitamin C when administered correctly during cancer treatment in combination with other agents can offer certain benefits and increase the chances of recovery.

Amygdalin, on the other hand, can only increase these chances to a very limited extent, since it would have to be administered in very high doses, which in turn would be accompanied by undesirable side effects. Thus, claims that these factors can heal cancer are also false. In principle, extreme caution is advised wherever recommendations are made for treating diseases using an alternative substance or method (such as pure juice fasting, GcMaf, or treatment with radionic devices)! Promises to cure cancer are usually not only objectively untenable and false, but also medically, ethically, and morally unjustifiable.

5.2 Implementation of Vital Field Therapy and Necessary Tumor Resolution

The twelve aspects of the vital field, which have already been outlined in this book, can provide a basic guide for effective complementary oncological treatment. The circle representing the twelve cancer-promoting factors and the twelve vital fields serves as a map for navigating the path toward health and recovery in order to achieve the goal of developing revitalizing self-healing powers (see figures 5 and 6 in the color insert). This is the most effective approach I can recommend for prevention against chronic diseases, including cancer. For the treatment of cancer, a basic course of treatment involving the twelve vital fields can be compared to rectifying the cause or causes of a basement flood. The leak(s) must be found and repaired so that no further water floods the basement. This does not mean that all the damage is immediately rectified; while the tumor that has grown on the tilted terrain of the human organism may not yet have been eliminated, another constant negative influence has been removed. Although treating the tumor in such a way that it shrinks (or, ideally, disappears) while taking care not to damage the terrain is a great challenge, it is possible with the help of vital field therapy.

"Primum Non Nocere"

The quote "first, do no harm" has been ascribed to Hippocrates (around 460–360 BC). In its more detailed version, the quote states that "in the case of an illness, one must take care of two things: Do good or at least do no harm."[8] In full, the quote reads as follows: "Primum non nocere, secundum cavere, tertium sanare," which translates as: "First, do no harm, second, proceed with care, third, heal."

In no other medical discipline is this concept more disregarded than in oncology. There is a general belief that doctors have no choice but to expose cancer sufferers to the severe side effects of established and generally accepted treatments. The question, however, is whether this is really expedient and necessary in every case.

In each individual case, the following questions must be addressed conscientiously, but also weighed up time and again: Which and how many of the treatments and their side effects does a patient have to accept? How often, for how long, and how intensively should standard treatments such as surgery, chemotherapy, radiation therapy, immunotherapy, or hormonal therapy be carried out, given the high risk of experiencing the severe side effects associated with them? How and at what price are patients provided the option of living longer with their disease and enjoying a good quality of life?

One of a doctor's most important tasks is to provide their patient with a comprehensive analysis of the relationship between the desired benefits and side effects of a proposed course of therapy. This generally takes a long time.

Treatments offered in accordance with guidelines can be supplemented or expanded in terms of their therapy options in many ways by using complementary or integrative medicine. When used in various combinations, these therapies can also strengthen conventional treatments (e.g., by using hyperthermia therapy), alleviate side effects (e.g., by using enzyme therapy), and improve quality of life (e.g., through mindfulness-based stress reduction). In certain cases, a doctor working in accordance with the principles of holistic medicine might decide together with their patient upon an individual course of therapy that goes beyond the guidelines, following well-considered reasoning based on evaluation of the individual case. In Germany, Austria, and Switzerland, it is possible to do this. In many other countries around the world, however, doctors are prohibited from taking this approach, as the respective legislature obliges them to follow the treatment guidelines in all cases and prohibits the use of alternative therapies.

I would like to highlight three types of therapy in particular that I consider to be *sophisticated* anticancer treatments because they have significant potential to eradicate cancer without causing the undesirable side effects associated with conventional treatments. These are known as insulin-potentiated therapy, photodynamic therapy, and partial or whole-body hyperthermia.

It is currently not known when these methods will be scientifically investigated and compared with conventional treatments on a large scale, so they are, in the best sense of the word, *complementary* medicine therapies. That is to say they are based on scientific models and documented observations but are not yet generally accepted as *standard*.

5.2.1 Insulin-Potentiated Therapy: How Sugar Can Destroy Cancer Cells

Insulin-potentiated therapy (IPT) is a safe and effective form of therapy that involves administering certain drugs under low-blood-sugar conditions.

For more than eighty-five years, this form of therapy has made a name for itself as a convincing method for treating cancer and chronic infections and is considered an alternative to chemotherapy with fewer side effects. It aims to attack cancer cells or chronically infected tissue (e.g., in the case of Lyme disease) in a very targeted manner and causes significantly fewer side effects than conventional therapies.

The advantage of this form of therapy is that specific medication such as anticancer drugs or antibiotics (antibacterial, antifungal, or antiviral agents) can be administered in low doses under insulin-induced low-blood-sugar conditions. In this way, side effects can largely be avoided, while the desired effect of the medication is intensified or even exponentiated.

ITP was developed in the 1930s by Mexican military doctor Donato Perez Garcia Sr. Since then, it has been used worldwide and been further refined and promoted by his grandson, Donato Perez Garcia Jr. I was able to learn the method from him and have been a certified member of the international academy for IPT since 2019.

The basis and functionality of IPT are as follows: Cancer cells have up to twenty times more receptors (binding sites) for insulin (the body's hormone for regulating blood sugar) on their cell surface than healthy cells. They are also primed for sugar utilization and take in ten to fifteen times more sugar per unit of time than healthy cells. IPT makes use of cancer cells' uptake of sugar by lowering blood sugar prior to administering anticancer drugs by around fifty to sixty milligrams per deciliter by injecting insulin intravenously. This is deliberately intended to trigger controlled low blood sugar (hypoglycemia) before a mixture of sugar and the required medicinal substance is injected in the same way. During the *sugar crisis* of low-blood-sugar levels, the cancer cells and chronically inflamed and infected cells open up their channels for the sugar they crave, and in doing so, "devour" the drug. This means a lower dose of the drug (10–30 percent of the regular dose) is enough to damage or kill the cells in question in a targeted way. IPT has few or no significant side effects and can be carried out for as long as is deemed useful or necessary to bring the disease under permanent control or force it into regression (remission).

Solid tumor diseases can be cured only rarely with standard orthodox chemotherapy. The general toxicity of the treatment, the inability of the treatment to specifically target cancer cells, and the numerous severe side effects on all healthy organs are some of the limiting factors of conventional treatments that affect the blood and immune cells in particular, but also have an adverse effect on the liver and put a lot of strain on the kidneys, digestive organs, and brain (hence the symptoms of "brain fog" and "chemo brain" described by those undergoing chemotherapy). Like conventional therapies, IPT can "cure" tumor-based diseases only in rare cases. What it can do, however, is help stop progressive diseases and reduce the tumor burden or bring it under control, thereby helping the patient to maintain a better quality of life. Doctors with experience in IPT therapy believe and understand how similar or better results can be achieved through this type of therapy than with regular-dose therapy, because the dose administered is so much lower and the drug targets cancer cells much more effectively. Here at the Arcadia practice, we offer IPT with both biological anticancer agents (such as turmeric extract, resveratrol, artemisia, vitamin C, and dichloroacetic acid) and standard orthodox chemotherapy in low doses. For us and our cancer patients, this represents a safe treatment option with few side effects, and we have been impressed by its efficacy.

5.2.2 Photodynamic Therapy: How Cancer Cells Can Be Killed with Light and Oxygen

Photodynamic therapy (PDT) is a new and particularly interesting variant of laser therapy for cancer treatment; it is carried out using a light-sensitive substance. Studies have shown that cancer cells have a special transport mechanism for chlorophyll through which they absorb more than sixteen times as much chlorophyll per unit of time as healthy neighboring cells do.

In PDT, an infusion is used to administer what is known as a photosensitizer (a light-sensitive substance) into the bloodstream, which is then specifically concentrated in tumor cells. One of the most effective photosensitizers is semisynthetic chlorin e6, which is made from a green dye known as chlorophyll. A pharmacological process removes part of the molecule from the chlorophyll obtained from grass, which changes the light-absorption behavior of the substance.

Three hours after the infusion is administered, a sufficient concentration level of the photosensitizer has accumulated in the tumor tissue and a laser fiber optic cable is inserted into the tumor tissue. The subsequent irradiation with laser light at a very specific wavelength activates the substance absorbed by the cancer cells in such a way that oxygen radicals are briefly formed through the formation of singlet oxygen molecules, which destroy the tumor cells. These oxygen radicals exist only for a few seconds before they break down again into normal oxygen. Because this substance does exactly what is expected of it in just a few seconds, which is to kill cancer cells before it transforms into harmless oxygen again, no toxins remain in the body.

The treatment takes effect less than half an hour after inserting the laser fiber-optic cable and does not cause any significant side effects.

Once the therapy session has been completed, it takes several weeks for the immune system to clear away the dead cancer cells and for the tumor to visibly shrink. It is essential for the patient to undergo a meticulous follow-up check after these weeks.

5.2.3 **Local or Regional Deep Hyperthermia**

Deep hyperthermia involves irradiation of the tumor using radio waves to trigger overheating of the tumor and thereby achieve synergies in combination with other procedures. Therapeutic use of heat is probably the oldest form of cancer therapy in the history of medicine. It is believed that even the ancient Egyptians burned out tumor wounds using a branding iron—a process described in a papyrus from the sixteenth century BC, which was discovered by American Egyptologist Edwin Smith in Luxor (Egypt) in 1862. Tissues are destroyed by caustic agents, or heat, in a process known as cauterization, which can also be used to stop bleeding.

Hippocrates was convinced that if cancer could not be cured by heat, then it was incurable. The healing power of fever (the body's very own "fire") is described in Hippocrates' *Aphorisms*. "The iron (scalpel) heals what medicines cannot. What iron cannot heal, fire heals, and what fire does not heal must be considered incurable." The following saying was also passed down to us from his teacher, Parmenides (circa 520–460 BC): "Give me the power to trigger a fever and I will cure any disease!"

Hyperthermia refers to a type of artificially induced fever and the therapeutic application of heat. It is used to overheat either the entire organism (whole-body hyperthermia) or part of it (local hyperthermia) under controlled conditions. Fever therapy triggers certain reactions in the whole organism, the immune system, or specifically in the tumor, which are very useful for treating cancer. These medical effects include triggering an immune modulation or "internal tumor vaccination." During this process, the heat causes cancer cells to form what are known as *heat shock proteins* on their surface. This makes them more "visible" to the immune system, which is then able to attack them. Hyperthermia treatments also create a clearly measurable synergy effect when carried out alongside radiation therapy. The cancer cells try to defend themselves against the radiation by initiating repair processes during and after ionizing or particle radiation treatment, which is one of the undesirable side effects of radiation therapy. In the worst-case scenario, some cancer cells "gain strength" and manage to emerge from radiation therapy stronger and more aggressive than before.

The heat generated by hyperthermia treatments, however, makes cancer cells sensitive to radiation treatment (such as classic radiation therapy using gamma rays) and blocks the repair processes of these cells, such that the destruction caused by the radiation is prevented from being hindered to a lesser extent. The effectiveness of a large number of anticancer drugs used in chemotherapy can be increased when administered in combination with hyperthermia treatments without increasing the number or severity of side effects that occur in healthy cells. The heat produces what is known as the "potentiation effect"; chemotherapy agents containing platinum, for example, have a much stronger effect when administered in combination with hyperthermia than they would at normal body temperature. The effect of new immunotherapy agents such as "checkpoint inhibitors" (e.g., nivolumab, pembrolizumab, ipilimumab) is also intensified by hyperthermia. Immune checkpoints are receptors on the membrane of T cells that regulate the organism's immune response. In other words, they serve as "instructions" for the immune system. Tumor cells can use these immune checkpoints to avoid being recognized by the immune system and "escape" it. Checkpoint inhibitors interrupt this connection to immune checkpoints so that the immune system can recognize degenerated cancer cells and fight them. Heat also drives the momentum of these drugs and therefore the overall effectiveness of the treatment. Blood circulation and the flow properties of the blood are improved by hyperthermia, which facilitates the transport of drugs into the tumor area (tumor perfusion), making this process more effective. Furthermore, the vitality of the immune cells is generally stimulated by hyperthermia, which is the purpose of fever: to improve the body's ability to fight inflammation and pathogens.

5.2.4 Local Radio Wave Hyperthermia: Local Application of Heat Therapy

We have been using various forms of hyperthermia in our practice since 2005. Local radio wave hyperthermia, which is applied exclusively to a single organ, or loco-regional hyperthermia, which is applied to an area of the body such as the pelvis or abdomen, is carried out over the course of one hour using a special device that sends radio waves at a frequency of 13.54 megahertz through the patient's body. During this process, two applicators (also called antennae) are placed parallel to each other on each side of the body in order to allow the radio wave field to flow through the body for an hour. The patient feels the area growing increasingly warm but does not experience any pain. Healthy tissues allow the radio waves at this frequency to pass through largely unhindered, and therefore only increase slightly in temperature. Tumor tissues from cancer cells absorb more energy in this frequency spectrum. According to physicists, the cancer cells' energy absorption is at its highest at this frequency. This causes them to overheat, creating conditions that are not ideal for them, and inducing the aforementioned effects.

Laboratory tests have also shown that these frequencies trigger a process known as apoptosis, which means some of the cancer cells exposed to the frequencies begin to die off naturally. In order to achieve the desired effects of the medical treatment, ten to fifteen treatments are carried out in the space of one hour. Ideally, they should be carried out alongside a parallel infusion or radiotherapy treatment. In our practice, each hyperthermia treatment session is accompanied by an infusion made up of the items listed in chapter 6, which are primarily biological anticancer agents.

5.2.5 Whole-Body Hyperthermia: Using Heat to Stimulate the Immune System

Another form of heat treatment is moderate, whole-body hyperthermia at temperatures between 39°C and 41°C (102°F and 105°F). This treatment was developed by New York surgeon William B. Coley (1862–1936), who in January 1883, treated a nineteen-year-old cancer patient for the first time with injections of febrile bacteria (a mixture of *Streptococcus pyogenes* and *Serratia marcesens*). The bedridden young man had an inoperable soft tissue mass measuring sixteen by thirteen centimeters, a sarcoma on the abdominal wall that had already penetrated the bladder and led to incontinence. Each of the bacteria injections administered triggered a fever reaction that increased the patient's body temperature to over 40°C. After four months, William B. Coley saw the disease go into complete remission. The young patient never experienced a relapse of the sarcoma and died of a heart attack twenty-six years later. A description of the case—which seemed almost like a miracle—was scientifically reviewed by Coley's niece, Helen Coley Nauts, alongside one thousand other treatment cases, many years after William B. Coley's death, and subsequently was documented in numerous publications. Coley himself worked on a textbook about fever therapy until shortly before his death, but the book was never completed or published. For over forty-four years, William B. Coley treated cancer patients with injections of bacterial mixtures at a time when antibiotics and effective antipyretic drugs were unavailable. In over 50 percent of over one thousand cases, he managed to stabilize patients or lead them into remission. It is a wonder that fever therapy for cancer has not garnered more attention. In most countries across the world, the active form of this procedure has long been banned. But why? Just a few years after Coley's death, fever therapy was discredited as old-fashioned and dangerous and gave way to the more "modern" methods of radiation and, later, chemotherapy.

The passive form of fever therapy experienced a revival, especially in Germany after World War II, largely thanks to two researchers: Stuttgart radiologist Martin Heckel (1926–2007) and Dresden scientist Manfred von Ardenne (1907–1997), both of whom are considered pioneers in the discipline. Martin Heckel suffered from the effects of poliomyelitis and began treating himself with an infrared whole-body hyperthermia device that he built in the 1950s. His muscle pain and mobility problems improved so significantly during this treatment that he presented his device to the German radiotherapy journal *Strahlentherapie* in 1960. In 1971, he set up his own hyperthermia treatment center, where he mainly treated patients with musculoskeletal system diseases, chronic inflammation, and cancer.

Manfred von Ardenne was a brilliant scientist who was granted his first patent in the field of electrical engineering at the age of sixteen. He was behind six hundred patented inventions, including the first television (1930) and the scanning electron microscope (1937). After many decades of working in electrical engineering and nuclear physics research, he began to dedicate himself to cancer research following a historical conversation with the founder and director of the Berlin Kaiser Wilhelm Institute for Cell Physiology, Otto Warburg (who won the Nobel Prize for Medicine in 1931). See section 3.4, "Oxygen, Breathing, and Cancer Growth," page 82, and section 6.1.5, "Optimal Oxygen Supply," page 189) for more details.

His whole-body hyperthermia device functions using water-filtered infrared A emitters, which emit long-wave infrared A rays that penetrate deep into the tissue, resulting in particularly effective deep heating without damaging the skin. Von Ardenne was the first to use and systematically research passive whole-body hyperthermia administered using a device specifically developed for the purpose. His treatment methods were met with great interest in Germany and were successfully applied in a clinical setting and scientifically investigated in Dresden and at the Greifswald University Clinic, among others. In the early 1970s, his whole-body hyperthermia method was also successfully used in a hospital in Friedrichshafen, Germany. Plans for a hyperthermia research institute in Friedrichshafen were underway but were eventually blocked by interventions by the German Cancer Research Center in Heidelberg, which favored chemotherapy.

Politics, money, and power games tragically thwarted any further clinical development of whole-body hyperthermia in Germany. This is why, to this day, the treatment can be found almost exclusively in practices of doctors specializing in complementary medicine.

In our practice, we use both Martin Heckel's and von Ardenne's devices and, in parallel to moderate whole-body hyperthermia, administer medical oxygen through a nasal cannula, infusions of biological anticancer agents, and most importantly, infusions of high-dose vitamin C (for details, see chapter 6). Administration of oxygen was also part of Manfred von Ardenne's systematic multistep cancer therapy, which makes cancer cells more sensitive to the effects of a drug while strengthening the healthy organism via short-term oxygen optimization.

The additional detoxifying effect of pyretotherapy (fever therapy) should not be underestimated, although this has not yet been extensively scientifically researched. During a full-body hyperthermia treatment, the patient sweats out hundreds of milliliters—and sometimes up to a liter—of sweat and receives corresponding amounts of pure, filtered water to compensate. A therapeutic water replacement takes place, which noticeably contributes to significantly better well-being after fever therapy. Fever therapy also has a detoxifying effect.

5.2.6 Fever and Mental Well-Being: Initiating the Mental Healing Processes

A phenomenon that has been largely neglected up until now and that I noticed from my early observations of patients before and after fever therapy, is a positive change in mood. Mental blockages, as well as a depressive mood in patients, both of which are common in oncology alongside anxiety and inner tension, are positively influenced by moderate fever therapy in a significant way. It is imperative for trained staff to accompany patients during the two to three hours it takes to administer the hyperthermia treatment. Not only must staff monitor the technical and medical implementation of the treatment, they should also support the patient through their fever experience and be there for them in the truest sense of the word, as the patient tells their life story, shares their grief, and often cries. Psychotherapists know how beneficial it can be for a patient to let go, acknowledge feelings, and cry during a therapeutic procedure. Before starting whole-body hyperthermia, we let our patients take a warm foot bath to enable them to mentally prepare for the treatment and to raise their body temperature. Once the fever therapy is complete, patients are asked to express their mood using colors.

————

Figure 7 (see the color insert) shows a typical example of two pictures—one created before and one after fever therapy on the same day. An image speaks a thousand words. What does each picture express? Which one represents chaos, which one harmony? Which one looks threatening, which one hopeful? The images were created spontaneously; the only stipulation was for the patient to express their mood intuitively and directly using colors. On the day after the fever therapy, our patients regularly report feeling relieved and revitalized, both physically and mentally. In our clinic, we call this area of work "psycho-thermo therapy."

5.2.7 Pulsating Magnetic Field Therapy: Treatments Using Pulsating Electromagnetic Frequencies

The healing properties of magnets have long been documented. It has been known since ancient times that our organism reacts to magnetism. Egyptian queen Cleopatra VII Philopator (69–30 BC) allegedly owned a magnetic headband, and Hippocrates of Kos is said to have treated patients with powdered magnetic stones. Paracelsus recommended the use of magnets for hemorrhoids or inflammation, while Viennese court physician Franz Anton Messner (1734–1815) caused a sensation with his spectacular treatment using magnets and his "magnetic hands," although given that his work increasingly focused on the latter, he would probably be considered as more of a hypnotherapist. The material and psychological elements of his treatments were completely intertwined, as was still customary in his day.

Modern pulsating electromagnetic frequency therapy (PEMF) has very little in common with its historical counterparts, but both acknowledge the fact that humans, like all life on earth, are susceptible to the effects of magnetic fields because we, too, have an electromagnetic nature. Without electromagnetism there would be no life.

Magnetism and electricity, the two elements that constitute electromagnetism, appear whenever charged particles move around an electrical conductor. This occurs in a bicycle dynamo, for example, as a result of the interaction between copper wires and the movement of the wheel, in a living cell between charged atoms (called ions), and in electrical conductors like the smallest protein tubes in an organism, known as microtubules, which give our cells their internal structure. Electromagnetism also exists in inanimate nature: on earth (as a result of the movements of its core) and elsewhere in the universe beyond our planet, wherever there is energy and matter in motion. In the 1970s, surgeon Fritz Lechner (1921–2013) and Munich physician Werner Krauss (1884–1959) developed a method for creating a positive effect on sick or damaged cells in the body with the help of pulsating magnetic fields. Initially, they primarily treated patients with broken bones and wounds that were difficult to heal—and with great success.

Given that every living cell (whether plant, animal, or human) has its own electromagnetic field, they can all be affected by electromagnetic fields to which they are exposed. This also means they can become damaged by electromagnetic fields, which is why the issue of electrosmog (emitted by high-frequency devices in our environment, in particular cell phones and transmitter masts) is becoming increasingly urgent. Gamma rays, which are particularly strong rays with an ultra-high frequency that kill cells by causing their molecules to explode, are used in radiation therapy.

In PEMF, an electronic device is used to generate a pulsating magnetic field of the order of between ten and eight hundred microtesla ("Tesla" is the unit of measurement for magnetic flux density named after Serbian physician Nikola Tesla). Most commonly administered at a frequency of around two hundred hertz (waves per second), these are relatively slowly oscillating magnetic fields that have a positive effect on the electrical conductivity of cells. By way of comparison, microwave ovens and cell phones oscillate at a frequency millions to billions of times faster, which explains the fact that they have a very different effect on biological systems such as humans.

The electromagnetic field used in PEMF therapy, which is also called magnetic therapy because of its relatively high magnetic field density, is directed through a cable into a therapy mat or pillow. The patient either lies down on the therapy mat or places the pillow on the part of the body to be treated to allow the pulsating magnetic fields to take effect on the body for a period of time. After a few minutes, the patient experiences a subtle, pleasant feeling of warmth, which is the result of improved blood circulation rather than the heat from the applicators (the pillow, mat, toroidal coils, or a stick, the latter of which is used for more precise application). The body's cells absorb the PEMF energy via induction, a process comparable to putting an electric toothbrush on charge. The duration of a therapy session is between ten and forty minutes and should be carried out several times, from a few times a week to twice a day, as required. One of the first and most important effects of the treatment is a significant improvement in the cells' oxygen uptake. This in turn benefits the energy metabolism of the entire organism, including its defense mechanisms.

Over decades, hundreds of scientific studies have proven that PEMF therapy has a measurable positive effect on many diseases. It has been proven to help broken bones heal faster, has positive effects on rheumatic joint diseases, improves wound healing, is used effectively in osteoporosis (bone atrophy), is helpful for stroke aftercare, has a pain-reducing effect, and improves kidney and liver function. The therapy has no known side effects.

The following scientifically documented effects have been observed in humans and summarized in specialized literature on PEMF:

- Strengthening of the skeleton through improved mineralization and processes that counter aging (anti-osteoporosis effect)
- Increased production of endorphins, the anti-pain hormones that our brains produce
- Improved sleep
- Increased ATP production in the mitochondria
- Improved oxygen supply and microcirculation
- Muscle relaxation and stress reduction
- Improved wound healing and tissue regeneration

5.2.8 **Does PEMF Therapy Also Help with Cancer?**

From the observations that have been made so far, it would appear that PEMF therapy can support many of the organism's important basic functions: improved blood flow (in particular microcirculation), improved oxygen uptake and saturation in tissues (and thus a significant counter action to cancer-promoting oxygen deficiency in tissues at risk of cancer, which is known as tissue hypoxia), optimization of the membrane charge of body cells (which can be clearly observed in live blood dark field microscopy before and after a single PEMF treatment), stimulation of the activity and mobility of white blood cells (the immune system), as well as an improvement of the detoxification function of cells and the organism as a whole. These effects are very useful, for both the prevention of cancer and keeping preexisting cases under control.

But are there any effects in addition to those described that specifically target cancer?

While only a few clinical studies have been carried out, these—as well as numerous tests on cancer cells—have already yielded remarkable results.

Cancer cells from human breast and colon cancer tumors have been intensively studied in laboratory conditions to examine how they react to PEMF. These studies have clearly demonstrated that PEMF has a direct growth-inhibiting effect on cancer. The most positive outcome is that this growth-inhibiting effect was observed only in cancer cells, leaving normal cells unharmed. In studies on mice, those that were implanted or injected with breast cancer cells showed an impressive (30–70 percent) reduction in breast cancer growth when treated with PEMF for up to six hours per day for a period of four weeks. Positive effects were also observed in mice with liver cancer and malignant melanomas.

As with all preclinical studies, the next challenge is of course to determine the circumstances under which this effect will occur, not only on cancer cells in petri dishes, but also in humans, and how exactly PEMF treatments should be carried out on cancer patients. Although clinical studies are available, no large, systematic, randomized, or double-blind studies have been carried out as required by standard clinical oncology. Unfortunately, this means there is no research funding or interest on a large scale, despite all the positive pilot studies.

In the available clinical studies, however, an overall positive effect was observed, and no side effects were clearly apparent. PEMF often relieves pain caused by cancer.

In a study published in 2005 on a group of forty-two patients with liver cancer for whom chemotherapy was deemed unsuitable, five patients reported a complete reduction of pain, and two further patients reported a significant reduction in pain, immediately after beginning PEMF therapy. In four cases, a partial decrease in tumor burden was observed, and in sixteen other cases, increased stability of the disease was documented, lasting for a period of over twelve weeks. The fact that these results have not led to further, larger-scale clinical studies being carried out is astonishing!

PEMF therapy is one of the therapies I have recommended most to patients over the past twenty years, whether to permanently improve biological terrain or to help keep cancer at bay alongside other therapies. The observations and positive experiences documented over the past two decades have given me reason to emphatically recommend this treatment. The precise methods for administering PEMF treatments are outlined in chapter 6.

Chapter Six

Cancer Therapies: Outside the Box

We cannot solve problems by using the same kind of thinking we used when we created them.

—ALBERT EINSTEIN

If a problem seems unsolvable, expand the framework. "Thinking outside the box" means being unconventional and creative, questioning the known limitations and thus incorporating all the essential criteria for problem solving. If you want to think *outside the box*, you have to know the box well. The content of this book so far is the basis for the practical therapies described in this chapter, from which you can choose the ones that are most suitable and feasible for you. This book aims to give you the tools to find a doctor or therapist whom you can trust and who will guide you in an experienced and competent manner to select and implement the therapies. Ideally, it is a doctor you already know or who is already looking after you. If this is not yet the case, my advice to you is: Don't be afraid to go in search of the right therapist for you!

In the following, many food supplements and natural remedies are mentioned and recommended that serve to increase the body's self-healing powers. I would like to explicitly point out here that I strongly recommend choosing the remedies and their dosages, which cannot always be specified in this book, together with experienced doctors. When it comes to the treatment of diseases, do not experiment on your own, but seek advice from an experienced doctor!

What is presented here is intended to provide a map and to make you aware of the treatment options that you can implement together with an experienced and trained doctor or therapist. The book and especially the contents of this chapter do not replace a textbook or training in naturopathy. However, it can provide an overview of possible therapies and give suggestions that will help you talk to your doctor or therapist with more awareness and with the right questions. It is also important to consider possible interactions with medicines you are already taking. Advising and monitoring the intake of all medicines and natural remedies belongs in the hands of an experienced doctor and should never be done on your own!

Now let's look at the *map* of the twelve vital fields again from the point of view of strengthening health, recovery, and healing. Each of these twelve fields can bring to our attention a specific nuance, a subject that we should consider for our recovery or caring for our health.

6.1 Outside-the-Box Therapies According to the Twelve Vital Fields

6.1.1 Inflammation Control and Inflammation Therapy

Not every inflammation is triggered by microorganisms. Often, it is also autoimmune reactions or a mixture of both that can lead to inflammation. To detect silent inflammation, blood and stool tests can be helpful.

Blood Test for Inflammatory Values

The measurement of the highly sensitive C-reactive protein (hsCRP) is ten times more sensitive than that of the "normal" inflammation parameter CRP. At values above 0.56, it already indicates a silent inflammation. Other blood values that can provide conclusions about silent inflammation are tryptophan, kynurenine, and antibodies of lipopolysaccharides, which are measured by special laboratories.

Inflammation Control

After treating the cause of one or more inflammations, inflammation control is the most important therapeutic measure. The most important agents for this are the following.

CURCUMIN

Turmeric extract (curcumin), when taken orally, acts almost exclusively in the intestine, as absorption through the intestinal mucosa is very low. For this reason, various products are provided with additives to increase the bioavailability at least somewhat. This is the case, for example, with piperine from black pepper, with curcumin oils, which work by encasing the curcumin in fat (liposomal curcumin), and with a carbohydrate coating. For direct use in the treatment of cancer, administration by injection promises the highest success.

PROTEIN-SPLITTING ENZYMES

Protein-splitting enzymes support inflammation control and have an anti-inflammatory effect. The proteolytic enzymes include, for example, bromelain from pineapple; papain from papaya; trypsin, chymotrypsin, and pancreatin from animal products; and proteases from specially cultivated mushrooms. Available in capsule form, they should be taken thirty to sixty minutes before meals in order to develop their anti-inflammatory function in the blood without first coming into contact with food in the stomach. Otherwise, they have only a digestive effect.

OMEGA-3 FATS

Omega-3 fats protect our cells and also have an anti-inflammatory effect. They work most effectively in the form of EPA and DHA from marine sources, such as krill or saltwater fish. For vegans, there are corresponding products made from algae. Furthermore, an anti-inflammatory diet should inherently be followed to control inflammation. PEMF therapy also has a positive effect on the organism in controlling inflammation.

6.1.2 Detoxification

Our organism has four toxin-removal pathways by means of which we can egest toxins that have been absorbed or have developed in us. Supporting these pathways is the basis of a healthy detoxification function.

Detoxification via the Intestine

Normally, a person has a bowel movement once or twice a day, at least every other day. Optimal is once or twice a day, with a formed consistency and without pain when going to the toilet. If this is not the case, there is a need for treatment. Constipation should in any case be improved by an appropriate change of diet, more fiber, and more liquids. In special cases, the administration of a laxative is necessary. Enemas are highly detoxifying. The best method for doing this is to use an irrigator, an enema vessel with a rubber tube and an end piece with a regulating tap, which can be bought in any pharmacy. The coffee enema according to Max Gerson is still a classic in naturopathic oncology, which can also be used to stimulate the liver to detoxify. The caffeine absorbed through the rectum from about two hundred to six hundred milliliters of normal strength coffee (preferably organic espresso roast) reaches the liver directly through the blood vessels of the enterohepatic circulation (i.e., the venous system running between the rectum and the liver), where it stimulates the activity of the detoxification enzymes of the cytochrome P450 family, which in turn can effectively break down toxins in the liver and excrete them with the bile. In addition, theophylline and theobromine contained in the coffee have an anti-inflammatory effect and dilate the blood vessels of the intestine, stimulating the flow of bile and the contraction of the gallbladder. This leads to the liberation of the liver from waste products and to the cleansing and reduction of inflammation of the mucous membrane of the rectum. The coffee enema is best carried out in the morning and can be used daily for weeks or even months to promote detoxification.

The following natural remedies are suitable to stimulate the liver to detoxify and self-regulate: milk thistle extract with the active ingredient silymarin, best taken in the evening, or in the case of severe toxin and/or liver stress also in the morning as well as the evening; MSM; selenium; and the anthroposophical herbal remedy Choleodoron (a mixture of celandine extract and turmeric); as well as dandelion extract and yarrow, mainly as tea.

Detoxification via the Skin

Proper sweating once or several times a week promotes not only the cardiovascular system, but also the body's own detoxification via the skin. Physical activities and applications that lead to sweating support detoxification, such as sauna applications—for example, a classic Finnish sauna or also a milder infrared sauna, which can be done at home with appropriate equipment. Brush massaging the skin stimulates blood circulation and lymph flow and thus also detoxification. It is best to massage in the morning after getting up, with an appropriate natural brush from the periphery of the arms and legs toward the heart.

Moderate whole-body hyperthermia (page 170) is the most intensive form of detoxification therapy that we perform in our practice. It can be performed once a week over a longer period of time.

Detoxification via the Kidneys

Detoxifying measures via the kidneys should start with proper fluid intake. Urine should be light yellow at least once a day and always clear. Teas that support the efferent urinary tract include horsetail tea (also botanically known as *Equisetum arvense*) with its high silica content. This has to boil for more than fifteen minutes so that the silica is dissolved from the hard stalks of the horsetail. PEMF therapy, especially via the kidneys, additionally stimulates the kidneys' circulation and thus their excretory function.

Detoxification via the Breath

Relaxed, slow, and deep breathing promotes oxygen–carbon dioxide exchange and in this way has a deacidifying and detoxifying effect, which is particularly beneficial when one is outside in fresh air.

Detoxification Promotion through Medication

THE PROCAINE-BASE INFUSION

The procaine-base infusion has a detoxifying and anti-inflammatory effect by improving the acid–base buffer. The procaine that is active in it was intensively studied by the Romanian cardiologist and geriatric scientist Ana Aslan (1897–1988) and used for the treatment of numerous chronic inflammatory diseases as well as an anti-aging agent in the "Aslan therapy." Procaine was also used as a local anesthetic for a long time. It also has a variety of effects on nerves, blood vessels, and tissues.

The Effects of Procaine in Detail
- Anti-inflammatory (beneficial in many chronic diseases)

- Lowers sympathetic tone by reducing adrenaline production (anti-stress effect)
- Anti-allergic through the reduction of histamine release

Procaine is mixed with the body's most important base, sodium hydrogen carbonate, and in this combination develops an excellent effect on the regulatory and detoxification processes of the human organism.

To prepare an infusion, mix 100 milliliters of 8.4 percent sodium hydrogen carbonate in 250–500 milliliters of 0.9 percent NaCl (physiological saline solution) with—depending on the symptoms and condition—2–10 milliliters of 2 percent procaine.

This infusion can be administered several times a week. A therapy cycle consists of ten infusions. Infusion time is about forty-five to sixty minutes.

SULFUR AS A DETOXIFYING AGENT

MSM and alpha lipoic acid are available as detoxifying natural substances, both in oral form in capsules or as infusion solutions, which are used in cases of severe stress on the liver or the nervous system (numbness or nerve pain), for example, after chemotherapy.

Detection and Detoxification of Heavy Metals

An examination of the blood for heavy metals by means of a whole blood analysis can give important information as to whether a special detoxification therapy with chelators should be carried out. This belongs in the hands of a doctor with experience in the field of toxicology and chelation therapy. A chelator such as DMSA or DMPS is an organic chemical substance that binds a toxic metal, for example, mercury or lead, and renders it harmless.

The complex topic of amalgam remediation and toxicology in the maxillofacial region can be outlined only briefly here. Amalgam fillings consist of up to 50 percent mercury, a strong toxin that is gradually released from the fillings in small quantities and thus enters the body. It mainly blocks the body's own sulfur-containing enzymes, which are then no longer able to do their job in the metabolic process. Most of the time, patients who have been exposed to mercury from dental amalgam complain of diffuse and unspecific symptoms: chronic fatigue, exhaustion, and diffuse neurological symptoms, which are sometimes severe and cannot be clearly attributed. By measuring mercury in whole blood and ruling out other causes for the symptoms, a tentative diagnosis can be made: chronic heavy metal exposure or even poisoning from dental amalgam.

In my experience, remediation of amalgam-filled teeth, if carried out carefully and professionally, leads to an increase in overall vitality. However, the remediation should be carried out only by dentists in cooperation with doctors who are experienced in the field of biological dentistry and detoxification therapies.

Detoxification through Adsorption to Minerals

ZEOLITE CLINOPTILOLITE

Zeolite clinoptilolite (ZC) is a microporous mineral of volcanic origin that occurs naturally all over the world in about one hundred different variations and belongs to aluminum silicates, that is, the siliceous minerals. Pharmacological processing into an ultrafine powder gives it a huge surface to which pollutants can adhere. This is called *adsorption* (from Latin *adsorptio* and *adsorbere*, meaning "to suck [in]"): the attachment and rendering harmless of toxins such as heavy metals. To put it simply, this mineral behaves toward heavy metals in our digestive tract like a sponge, which absorbs the toxins into its internal channels and releases sodium, potassium, or magnesium (ion exchangers). Overall, according to the latest research, ZC is also thought to have detoxifying, anti-inflammatory, and antioxidant effects.

The intestine does not absorb ZC itself nor the harmful substances bound to it, but releases them completely with the bowel movement. Among other things, this has positive effects on leaky gut (see section 3.5, "Maintaining Intestinal Health," page 89), confirmed in 2015 in a placebo-controlled double-blind study on fifty-two subjects.

Zonulin was measured in the stool as a marker for leaky gut syndrome. After three months of taking 1.85 grams of ZC daily, the initially elevated zonulin values fell by 30 percent into the normal range. To avoid interactions with other medicines, these should be taken at least two hours before taking the zeolite, which is best taken in the evening. While taking zeolite, make sure you drink enough fluids! When choosing an appropriate product, as with anything else, pay attention to the quality. There are reports of such products being contaminated with impurities and therefore completely failing in their detoxification-promoting task.

6.1.3 Nutritional Deficiencies and Food Supplements

In principle, an examination of vitamin, mineral, and micronutrient requirements should be carried out—as far as this is possible and reasonable in terms of expense—before treatment with food supplements. For the nutritional deficiencies known in large parts of the world, such as vitamin D_3 and selenium, but also for iron (especially for women of menstruating age) and zinc, this can be done easily and at low cost. Deficiencies should be compensated for by targeted treatment with the help of appropriate substances. Depending on gender and tumor type, between 30 percent and 90 percent of those affected follow this recommendation, often without the treating oncologist knowing. However, there are still no clearly defined maximum or reference values for most essential substances. Instead, there are values for the absolute minimum amount, the recommended daily intake, the recommended daily allowance, and—especially in nutritional medicine circles—the optimal daily intake.

Vitamin D_3

Let's take vitamin D_3 as a well-known example of how a vitamin D deficiency brings with it a 30–50 percent higher risk of developing, for example, colon, breast, or prostate cancer.

Table 6.1 shows the interpretation of different concentrations of the biologically active form of vitamin D_3 in micrograms (μg) per litre (L) of blood.

There are similar tables for many of the approximately ninety substances that we need to live. Orthomolecular medicine deals with those substances that are naturally present in the body and on which it depends. These include vitamins, minerals, trace elements, amino acids, and essential fatty acids, which should be present in sufficient quantities to keep the organism healthy. However, please do not experiment; instead, seek the advice of an expert!

Only an experienced doctor, therapist, or nutritionist can use their knowledge and collection of literature to ensure an optimal supply of essential nutritional building blocks and, if necessary, also prescribe therapeutic doses of a nutritional substance in the sense of orthomolecular medicine. Only

Table 6.1. Interpretations of D$_3$ Concentrations in Blood

Vitamin D$_3$ value in the blood in µg/L	Interpretation
<5	Most severe vitamin D deficiency
5–10	Severe vitamin D deficiency
10–20	Vitamin D deficiency
20–30	Lower normal range
30–50	Good vitamin D level
50–100	Upper normal range, achievable only by substitution
100–150	Overdosed substitution
>150	Vitamin D intoxication

they can assess and accurately evaluate the values of their patients measured in the laboratory with regard to their respective disease situation and the other treatments, so that the respective substances have a desired therapeutic effect in correspondingly high doses. Examples of this are selenium or vitamin C, vitamin D or iodine, which in higher doses have specific effects that go beyond those of a food component. In my experience, the basic supply of such substances, which people in Western industrialized countries are regularly lacking and whose concentration could or should be optimized by taking food supplements, includes omega-3 fatty acids, vitamin D$_3$ (especially at the darker time of year!), vitamin C, selenium, zinc, iodine, magnesium, and boron. Their content in our food has greatly decreased, due to, among other things, the consequences of modern agriculture, and therefore it has also decreased in our organism.

For women from the onset of menstruation onward, iron is a very common deficiency that should be checked and, if necessary, supplemented. Anemia due to iron deficiency is considered a possible risk factor for breast cancer!

On the other hand, an excess of iron is a risk factor for colon cancer, which is why the consumption of red meat contributes to health only in moderation, while regular consumption of red meat increases the risk of developing colon cancer. Anemia due to iron deficiency should therefore be treated and red meat should be consumed only in moderation, at most 150 grams per day once or twice a week.

The officially recommended amounts or doses of food supplements are calculated for healthy adults. As soon as a person takes one or more medicines, the need for vitamins, minerals, and essential fatty and amino acids changes significantly. This is of particular importance for cancer patients: They are sometimes treated with very strong drugs and medicines with many side effects, usually over a long period of time.

Iodine—an Important Trace Element

Iodine is a vital trace element not only for the thyroid gland but for the entire organism, and must be ingested in sufficient quantities through the diet. The word *iodine* comes from the ancient Greek and means "violet," because iodine, which shines dark grey in its solid state, evaporates as a violet gas when heated. Iodine, which is important for all body cells and especially for the mammary glands, can be measured safely only in urine samples. This is not a routine examination and constitutes a special effort that is rarely implemented. Nevertheless, iodine deficiency is quite widespread, especially in people living in areas far from the coast.

The approximately fivefold lower incidence of breast cancer in Japan is explained by the adequate iodine supply there due to the traditional fish- and seafood-rich diet of Japanese people. For large parts of the world, there is a lack of iodine in the soil because the glaciers of prehistoric times washed away the naturally occurring iodine. Iodine occurs naturally mainly in marine life forms such as fish, algae, and seafood, which, on average, we Western land-bound cultures do not consume enough of in our diet. The result is an epidemic iodine deficiency, which current studies link to the rapid rise in breast cancer in particular. For all those who do not regularly eat fish or seafood, my recommendation for adults is to make sure they have a daily iodine supply of at least 200 micrograms. Pregnant women and nursing mothers need slightly more (about 260 micrograms). The use of iodized salt should be standard for everyone. It contains 15 to 25 micrograms of iodine per kilogram of salt, which means the average 5 grams of salt we eat per day contains about 75–125 micrograms of iodine. Women with breast disease, from mastopathies with cysts to breast cancer, may benefit from iodine supplementation or treatment, which involves much higher daily doses of iodine. Whether and how much iodine is supplemented should always be discussed with an experienced physician. A simple and extremely inexpensive source of iodine is *Lugol's solution*, which is a mixture of elemental iodine, potassium iodide, and water. One drop of the 5–9 percent solution diluted in a glass of water will definitely cover the daily iodine requirement. However, this should be implemented only if autoimmune thyroid disease with hyperfunction has been ruled out.

The Physiological Importance of Iodine

It is known that iodine is the decisive building block for the vital thyroid hormones T3 and T4. Our body therefore stores some of the iodine ingested with food in the thyroid gland in order to then incorporate it into the hormone-active molecule. Our entire metabolism is regulated by these iodine-containing thyroid hormones. This includes not only the oxygen consumption and energy balance of the cells, but also the function of our cardiovascular system and digestive tract, as well as the development of the brain and cognitive development in unborn babies and children.

For the issues of "cancer prevention" and "treatment," it is of particular importance that the female body also absorbs iodine in the mammary glands and stores it as a depot to supply to the child during breastfeeding.

A good iodine supply is therefore particularly important because thyroid hormones control and influence numerous functions in our organism. According to the latest findings, this also includes the control of apoptosis (cell death), especially in glandular cells: The binding of iodine to special fats (lipids) in the mammary glands produces the iodine lactones, which influence cell growth and differentiation processes and initiate natural cell death.

The influence of iodine on mammary gland growth has been studied in medical circles for fifty years. Iodine lactones can (partially) inhibit pathological breast tissue, such as cystic and cancerous gland growth, and induce apoptosis of pathological cells. Iodine thus becomes an important trace element for breast health. In addition, iodine has a high antioxidant potential, because the neutralization of oxygen radicals, for example, in glandular tissues, makes iodine a nutritional substance with great preventive significance, including with regard to other diseases caused by civilization, such as arteriosclerosis or cataracts (clouding of the lens). Further areas of application for the use of iodine are protection against autoimmune diseases and fatigue (exhaustion syndrome) or their treatment.

6.1.4 Treating and Drinking Fresh Water

As described in section 3.3, "Water: An Elixir of Life," page 78, drinking fresh, pure water is the basis of our life. Today, we have a number of devices at our disposal to improve the quality of drinking water. Since hardly anyone has direct access to fresh, uncontaminated spring water, it makes sense to buy a water filter or a water swirler. In our practice, we offer our patients both ultrapure water from a reverse osmosis system and swirled water.

Under the keywords "drinking water swirler" or "reverse osmosis" for home use, you can find a lot of information today that you can use to make your choice. If you live in a house or apartment with polluted drinking water quality (the local waterworks will provide a drinking water analysis on request), you can consider installing a filter or reverse osmosis system. The result is usually noticeable: Pure water is "easier" to drink in that it immediately creates the feeling of wanting to drink a little more and with pleasure. The immediate sensation in the mouth is also much lighter and tastier than with other waters. Pure water, rid of harmful substances, transports the substances dissolved in it better into the cells and dissolves the substances to be excreted better for the upcoming detoxification.

In my household, I have been using drinking water swirlers for thirty years and start every day with a large glass (about three hundred milliliters) of fresh, swirled water. This not only compensates for the loss of fluids during the night, but at the same time stimulates excretion and invigorates the entire organism. I know of no other health-promoting measure that is so beneficial and brings about such a great and immediate increase in well-being. Try it out!

6.1.5 Optimal Oxygen Supply

Spend more time in nature, go for walks, and learn to breathe more deeply and calmly. Create an exercise plan for yourself, depending on your age and performance level. My own experience is that long walks in the wood for one to several hours are of enormous benefit; they reduce stress, promote sleep, aid weight control, improve digestion and the flow of thoughts, and much more. Physical activity has been shown to be beneficial to health, in particular in the case of cancer, when practiced regularly, with breaks and adapted to one's ability. In Kelly Turner's book *Radical Hope*, sports activity is presented in detail as the tenth factor for "radical remissions," with numerous examples.

PEMF therapy (see section 3.4, "Oxygen, Breathing, and Cancer Growth," page 82) and infrared saunas increase blood flow and thereby also the oxygen supply to our organs. Both forms of therapy can easily be carried out regularly at home with the appropriate equipment. In the case of cancer in the chronic stage, I advise my patients to do both: daily treatment with PEMF, and home treatment with infrared devices several times per week.

6.1.6 **Maintaining Intestinal Health**

The best basis for planning and carrying out intestinal remediation is a thorough examination of the microbiome. Until a few years ago, investigations were based on the cultivation of intestinal bacteria and subsequent analysis of the quantity and composition of the bacterial strains grown under laboratory conditions. Today, it is the microbiome examination based on genetic analysis that represents the gold standard. This eliminates the problem that not all bacteria that live in our intestines grow and can be detected in the laboratory. The stool sample sent in for this examination is completely homogenized for the new diagnosis based on gene analysis and then examined for all the genes it contains. This gene analysis makes it possible to detect not only a much larger number of bacterial species, as well as their quantity and composition, but also fungi, yeasts, and parasites.

The multipage analysis result provides the doctor or therapist with a detailed representation of the entire microbiome, from which the therapy can be planned. In addition, a stool examination can provide important information about possible inflammations in the intestine, mucosal damage, or the presence of a leaky gut, by determining calprotectin and zonulin.

In addition to the treatment options with specific medicines for intestinal inflammations—for example, with a combination preparation of substances from myrrh, chamomile, and coffee charcoal, with dietary fibers from, for example, acacia fibers and with butyric acid from clarified butter (cooked butter, also called ghee)—pre- and probiotics, containing nutrients for good intestinal bacteria, are key for health in the organism. Bacterial mixtures with abundant physiologically important, health-promoting intestinal bacteria (in the range of 10^9 to 10^{10} bacteria per capsule) are also a good therapeutic agent. Similarly, aloe vera extracts or the juice of the plant have an effect that is anti-inflammatory and protects the intestinal mucosa.

As a rule, these remedies should be taken for three months and the result should preferably be evaluated on the basis of a second microbiome test.

6.1.7 Stress Reduction: Regaining the Psychoemotional Oscillation Capacity

Of all the stress reduction methods we can read about today, *mindfulness training* or *mindfulness-based cognitive therapy* (MBCT), often also called *mindfulness-based stress reduction* according to Jon Kabat-Zinn, seems to me to be one of the best. The method has been scientifically studied and found to be effective for depression, anxiety, and a range of psychological stress disorders that we all have at times to a greater or lesser extent. MBCT combines breathing and physical exercises with seven principles of awareness, which are:

- nonjudgmental thinking
- nonstriving
- accepting what is
- letting go
- being unprejudiced
- patience
- trust

For a better understanding, here is a short summary of these seven principles from the book *Full Catastrophe Living*, by Jon Kabat-Zinn.

Nonjudgmental Thinking. Be an impartial witness to your experiences. Observing without judging helps you to see what is in your awareness without intellectually influencing your perception or losing yourself in biased thoughts.

Nonstriving. There is no goal other than being yourself. It is not about achieving anything else, such as relaxation or enlightenment. Be yourself.

Accepting What Is. Be willing to see things as they are. By accepting what each moment in your life brings, you become able to live your life more *fully*.

Letting Go. Learn to let go of thoughts, ideas, things, events, desires, beliefs, hopes, and experiences, both pleasant and unpleasant. Allow things to be exactly as they are without becoming entangled in attachment or repulsion. Observing your breathing, feeling how you breathe in and out, is a good *anchor* to bring your consciousness into the now.

Being Unprejudiced (Unbiased and Curious Like a Child). Free yourself from expectations based on memories from the past. Observe how the moment unfolds, without any preconceived program, just in the presence of the present. Use your breath to bring your attention into the now.

Patience. Remember that all things take time. This is the alternative attitude to the restlessness of our inner impatience. Don't let your fears or desires for a particular outcome interfere with the quality of the moment.

Trust. Trust yourself and your feelings. Practice a sense of inner certainty that things will unfold in a reliable way, according to their nature.

Another method for regaining inner balance that I would highly recommend is learning and practicing heartfelt forgiveness. We all carry around memories of situations in which we felt unfairly treated, perhaps even cheated or abused. The desire, on the one hand, not to become bitter about it and to get rid of the baggage at some point, and on the other hand, to keep what happened alive in memory as a witness to the deep hurt, builds up an inner tension that usually makes forgiveness impossible for a long time.

In 2007, I became aware of a book titled *Radical Forgiveness*. After reading it intensively, I sought out the therapy and training center where the author, Colin Tipping, an English hypnotherapist, teaches and passes on his forgiveness method. In 2007–2008, I was trained as a coach of this method. Since then, I have been incorporating the forgiveness method into my discussions with our patients or recommending it to them.

This is a different, a complete forgiveness, out of the inner insight that everything that happens is, on a higher level, an effect of what has occurred before and strives toward a balance. To resist this seems pointless within this way of looking at things. If one surrenders to the "big picture" of events and becomes aware of the significance for one's own biography, a deep understanding can develop and a real acceptance can come about. Through this acceptance, it is even possible to feel gratitude. Humility and happiness are often part of this feeling. This complete forgiveness out of inner insight is paired with the undisguised acceptance that, after recognition and admission, radiates a serene calm that broadens the inner spaces and can reveal new paths with new strength.

It sounds banal to try to summarize this forgiveness in a few sentences, and yet it can change a biography or the course of one's life if one acquires this inner attitude of awareness. You can learn exactly how to do this in Tipping's book, by being coached by those trained in it, or in workshops and seminars. It is actually quite simple, but it still often needs a push from outside or some help to be able to make the change of perspective. From my own experience and from working with many patients over the last thirteen years, I can confirm that the Tipping method can have an amazing healing effect on health and the course of illness. Forgiveness heals.

In my experience, not only stress reduction but also a fulfilled life includes activities in which I can express myself as I am and which immediately give me the feeling that I am alive. This can be experienced or practiced, for example, in activities such as painting, dancing, making music, singing (in a choir or alone), pottery (and other craft activities such as weaving, spinning, sewing, carving, woodturning, sculpting, forging, and many more), poetry, writing, and playing. In this respect, there are no limits to creativity.

These activities create meaning as I experience them, simply because I want to do them and because I can. Some people shy away because they have the idea that these activities could turn you into an egoist, but the danger of this happening is extremely small among the people with a cancer diagnosis whom I have met as a doctor. However, the fear of this exists for many, because feeling free and being free are often unfamiliar. We can practice it a little every day, and grow every day.

6.1.8 **Discover and Transform Unhealthy Beliefs**

Another method to reduce stress is to find and change unhealthy beliefs. It comes from cognitive behavioral therapy and was developed by various psychotherapists in the 1960s–1980s. It is based on philosophical ideas that go back to the time of the ancient philosophers (Cicero, Seneca, Epictetus, and other Stoics).

In his courses, the American consultant radiologist and oncologist Oscar Carl Simonton placed great emphasis on a six-step exercise.

Step One

Take a piece of paper and write down a thought or a certain statement that causes you discomfort or stress.

- Ask yourself what assumption leads to the meaning or background of this thought/statement, and write this down under the stress-inducing thought.
- Repeat this process until you have arrived at a final basic assumption, which you also write down.
- While doing this, follow your feelings and not your intellectual mind.

This usually results in four to six sentences, the essence of which is a conviction that you yourself instinctively and unconsciously assume. This belief is the crux of the matter and creates discomfort and stress, which can have an effect from the unconscious, psychological level to the physical level.

Example:
Whenever something hurts, I think it could be a new cancer metastasis.
The new cancer metastasis will cause me more and more pain and rob me of my sleep.
Since all the treatments so far have not prevented it, it was probably all for nothing and I will die soon.
I have done everything wrong and I am ashamed that I will be abandoning my family soon when I die.
It is all my fault.

Identifying this (or any) set of unhealthy beliefs and having the courage to write them down is the most difficult part of the exercise. Most people need the help of a therapist or a coach.

Step Two

The second part of this exercise is to ask yourself the following questions for each of the sentences you have written down.

> Do I feel good when I think or read this sentence?
> Does this sentence support my health, my healing, my treatments?
> Does my stress decrease when I read and think this sentence?
> If I think this sentence long enough and repeat it over and over again, does it make anything better in my life?
> Is this sentence true? Would my best friend confirm that this sentence is true?

If you can answer no to three or more of these five questions, you can be sure that the sentence or sentences represent unhealthy beliefs. Unhealthy attitudes and beliefs are unhealthy because they are not "true" and disturb the inner, mental coherence experience and thus also the coherence of the organism, consciously or unconsciously.

Step Three

In the next step, please ask yourself the question: Do I want to continue to live with these unhealthy beliefs/attitudes?

If you can answer *no* to this question, go on to step four: changing the unhealthy attitudes.

Step Four

You could, for example, break down and change the above sentences as follows (do this in writing as well).

> When something hurts, I go back to what has helped me before. I
> make myself a hot water bottle, do a little gymnastics exercise, do a

breathing exercise, meditate, and feel how this makes the pain ease. If
it's a new metastasis, then I'll talk to my doctor and get examined.

I trust that I will get an effective treatment that I can adapt or change
from time to time. I trust that I can recharge my "batteries" while I
sleep and that my energy levels will improve again, no matter how
long I sleep.

I choose to continue those treatments that I believe will help me live my
life well and long. I know that my life on earth, like all other life, is
finite, and I am at peace with that.

I recognize the huge efforts I have already made and achievements that
I have already accomplished with this challenge of cancer. And I
am aware of the appreciation and love of my family and friends. I
welcome them into my life.

I drop all thoughts of guilt that I sometimes feel in connection with my
illness. I recognize that my life, as it is, is worth living and is mine. I
love my life, and I feel that my life loves me just as I am.

Step Five

Let these new thoughts pass through your soul in peace. Then ask yourself
the five test questions from step two again: How do you feel when you per-
mit the new thoughts? Better? Then choose these, and exchange the old ones
for the new ones!

Step Six

The sixth part involves the regular practice of the new healthy beliefs. Carry
the negative sheet (step one) folded up with you and read the old, unhealthy
beliefs whenever you notice that you have fallen back into that way of thinking. Say to yourself: "Ah, there you all are again, I know you well, you are
unhealthy beliefs. I am letting go of you now."

Then read the new, positive and healthy sentences from step four, aloud if
possible. These new sentences then become affirmations that help you think
what feels good. They reduce your stress, support your recovery or your life
with cancer, and are also true.

I have done this exercise hundreds of times with my patients and have
always witnessed how much physical strength and zest for life it releases. The

difficulty, however, is that this exercise works only if you do it regularly—daily and for at least one or two weeks.

6.1.9 Insulin and Blood Sugar Regulation

In addition to the dietary advice presented in section 3.2, ""Healthy Nutrition and Health-Promoting Dietary Supplements Using the Example of the Twelve Vital Fields," page 36, and in section 3.7, "Sugar: Cancer Driver of the First Order," page 108, the following means are suitable for optimizing blood sugar and the associated metabolic consequences.

- Berberine (a plant ingredient from *Berberis sargentiana*) has an anti-inflammatory effect and can be used to lower blood sugar and cholesterol levels.
- Cinnamon as a spice or aqueous cinnamon bark extract in capsule form lowers the blood sugar level and also has a positive effect on regulating blood lipids.

The essential trace element chromium, found for example, in chromium picolinate, an organically bioavailable chromium compound, is a cofactor of the hormone insulin and stimulates the absorption of sugar into the body cells. It can thus be used to regulate blood sugar. The daily recommended amount of chromium to be taken is between thirty and one hundred micrograms. Together with other substances (amino acids and a B vitamin), chromium forms glucose tolerance factor (GTF). The chromium content in the blood can be determined by a whole blood analysis and, if necessary, balanced by additional intake.

Dietary fibers (e.g., a mixture of acacia fibers, linseed, chia seed, psyllium, inulin, and healing clay) slow down the rise in blood sugar, among other things, and thus prevent rapid fluctuations in blood sugar and the subsequent increase in insulin secretion.

Intermittent fasting (eating within eight hours, for example, from midday to 8 p.m.) followed by sixteen hours of fasting (8 p.m. to midday) or skipping a main meal also has a positive effect on healthy blood sugar and insulin regulation.

6.1.10 **Optimizing the Immune System: Injection Therapy with Mistletoe Extracts**

In addition to the methods already mentioned, which relieve the immune system and strengthen it in its cancer-controlling and balance-creating function, there is a naturopathic form of therapy that can look back on a hundred years of practical application and can thus be counted among the classics of naturopathic oncology. According to recent studies, 40–80 percent of patients in Germany, Austria, and Switzerland also use complementary forms of therapy in addition to the established conventional medical methods for gynecological cancer.

Injection therapy with mistletoe extracts is the most widespread, both in adjuvant therapy (supplementary or supportive therapy measures, for example, after an operation as a follow-up treatment and as secondary-preventive therapy) and in the palliative stage of the disease.

This therapy goes back to the Dutch physician Ita Wegman and the Austrian philosopher and polymath Rudolf Steiner, who applied and taught it in the 1920s within the anthroposophical medicine they developed. Mistletoe injection therapy is now one of the most commonly used supplementary treatments for cancer in German-speaking countries. It has also been used for decades in the treatment of other chronic diseases for immunomodulation.

Among more than one thousand different components, mistletoe most notably contains the pharmacologically relevant ingredients mistletoe lectins and viscotoxins. These have a growth-inhibiting effect on cancer cells in cell cultures even in low doses and stimulate apoptosis; in other words, they have a redifferentiating effect and reactivate natural cell death. The ingredients of mistletoe also work synergistically with other conventional cytostatics.

Studies have also clearly shown that mistletoe extracts stimulate or modulate the immune system. Numerous randomized and nonrandomized controlled clinical trials have shown a positive influence on both survival time and quality of life in patients with gynecological tumors. Mistletoe injection therapy should be carried out by a doctor who has experience with it, and it is administered by injections under the skin (usually three times a week) over several months with breaks in between. Depending on the stage of the disease, this treatment may be given for years. To obtain optimal immunomodulation, the amount administered is slowly increased with gradual low doses. If, for example, there are metastases in the abdominal cavity or the pleura, the injection of high doses of mistletoe extract into body cavities such as the abdominal cavity is a special form of application. In high doses and intravenous applications, mistletoe extract can also have a direct cancer-killing effect, a cytostatic or cytotoxic effect. In parallel with chemotherapy, mistletoe therapy can significantly reduce chemotherapy's side effects.

Vital Mushroom Extracts and Adaptogens in Complementary Oncology

The vital mushrooms, whose collective name derives from the contents, include various varieties and species whose intake in the form of extracts has enjoyed growing popularity among cancer patients for several years. The Society for the Science of Vital Mushrooms (Gesellschaft für Vitalpilzkunde e.V) offers extensive and reliable information on this topic.

Vital mushrooms contain a wealth of vital substances and have been used for many years in the complementary treatment of cancer diseases, mainly because of their regulative effects on the immune system. Especially in the case of diseases in which the immune system no longer reacts in a targeted manner (as is the case with cancer), an immune-system-regulating treatment with vital mushrooms is an option.

The polysaccharides found in these mushrooms (for example, beta glucans) have the following effects, among others: They stimulate the fat metabolism and thus have a positive effect on cardiovascular diseases, they promote digestion, they have an immunomodulatory effect by activating and stimulating the maturation of defense cells, they have an activating effect on macrophages (phagocytes) and NK cells (natural killer cells) as well as on the formation of antibodies. Particularly in combination with enzyme preparations (especially proteases), vital mushrooms, especially shiitake and maitake mushrooms, prove to be good companions, especially before and during chemotherapy.

Adaptogenic Substances

Adaptogens are substances that positively regulate the stress response of our nervous system and immune system.

One of the best-known adaptogens, not only in cancer medicine, is cannabidiol (CBD) from *Cannabis sativa*. CBD works by regulating the natural endocannabinoid system (ECS), the body's own production and regulation of cannabis-like natural substances in our organism, the cannabinoids. The ECS is a primary regulatory system of our organism with messenger substances and corresponding receptors in almost all organs. It regulates sleep, appetite, pain, inflammation, memory, mood, and sexual behavior, among other things. The first cannabis receptor in our body cells, CB-1, was discovered in 1988. It is found mainly in the central nervous system. The second, CB-2, which acts in the immune system, was discovered in 1993. Our organism constantly produces these cannabis-like cannabinoids, with which it tries to adapt to the needs of our lives and keep stress levels in balance. Unfortunately, this endogenous system is less and less able to keep up with the increasing needs of our stressful lives. In addition, we often produce too many enzymes that reduce the positive effect of endocannabinoids. The cannabis plant contains up to one hundred different forms of cannabinoids, of which CBD and tetrahydrocannabinol (THC) are the best known. They can be used to positively influence the ECS when it is out of balance.

Some studies, especially preclinical studies on tissues and cells, have also been pointing to a possible cancer growth-inhibiting effect of CBD for at least ten years. Larger studies are desirable here, which could help us understand this effect even better and clarify unanswered questions about it. CBD is not addictive and has no intoxicating effect, as opposed to the well-known intoxicating cannabis substance THC.

THC can be prescribed by a doctor on a narcotic prescription and is now well described in science-based oncology. However, treatment with this substance should be carried out by a doctor who has experience with this form of treatment. THC has many effects that can be used especially in advanced forms of cancer: It has pain-relieving, anxiety-relieving, appetite-enhancing, and antispasmodic effects. For adults who have not had any experience with it in adolescence, it is assumed that THC is not addictive, which means that it can be discontinued at any time without producing abstinence symptoms. A mixture of THC, CBD, and cannabis terpenes, a pharmaceutically controlled cannabis extract, provides patients suffering from the late effects of cancer with an effective means of better managing the many symptoms, also in combination with synthetic painkillers. The subject of interactions with other medicines should also be discussed with a doctor so that the advantages and disadvantages can be weighed up individually in order to find the right dose and combination for the sufferer.

In addition to Siberian ginseng and *Rhodiola rosea*, I would like to highlight the extract of the Indian sleeping berry (botanically known as *Withania somnifera*), which has become known under the Sanskrit word *ashwagandha*, as another adaptogenic plant substance. The plant is called the queen of Ayurvedic herbs. Its extracts counteract the aging processes in our organism (anti-aging effect), reduce undesirable stress reactions and inner restlessness, and increase physical and mental performance. When taken in conjunction with physical exercise, it can improve the development of muscle strength.

6.1.11 Mitochondrial Medicine

The central role of mitochondria for our health, their importance for our life and the development or prevention of cancer has already been presented. Here are some practical tips to keep the mitochondria "fit."

Sports and Physical Exercise

All physical activities that are good for the heart, including walking and jogging, are beneficial.

Cold Training

Cold stimuli not only make mitochondria strong, but can also help them multiply: Alternating hot and cold showers, saunas followed by cold water showers, or Kneipp treatments with cold water have a very beneficial effect.

Altitude Training

Altitude training with inhalation therapy and alternating oxygen concentrations strengthens the cellular power plants. Intermittent hypoxia–hyperoxia therapy with special devices should be administered on at least ten different days, either daily or at least two to three times a week, for one hour each time, in order to achieve a noticeable effect. Such treatment cycles can be carried out several times a year.

Orthomolecular Medicine

Mitochondrial function can be supported by the use of high doses of vitamins, minerals, and trace elements. The following naturally occurring substances, which are also available in capsule form, have become particularly well known for their mitochondria-activating properties.

Coenzyme Q10 promotes the provision of mitochondrial energy for our active body cells in a complex way. Its positive effect, especially on the heart muscle, is scientifically well documented.

PQQ (pyrroloquinoline quinone) is a substance that we get about 0.1–1.0 milligrams of per day with food. Parsley, green tea, fruit—especially kiwis and papayas—spinach, and fermented soybeans such as natto or miso are particularly rich in PQQ. Babies get PQQ from breast milk. PQQ also supports the complex processes of the mitochondria in the production of energy.

L-carnitine primarily improves the burning of fat in the mitochondria and thus their energy production.

Pulsed electro-magnetic field therapy, PEMF (see chapter 5), has a stimulating effect—as does everything else that reduces chronic ("silent") inflammation, strengthens the microbiome, remedies nutritional deficiencies, and reduces toxin loads—and also strengthens the basic function of our billions of mitochondria.

6.1.12 Optimize the Acid–Base Balance: Naturopathic Deacidification Therapy

In addition to the treatments described in sections 3.2 (on nutrition) and 3.3 (on water), we use the following therapeutic methods to balance or optimize the acid–base balance (ABB).

Circulation and Oxygen Supply

Here, too, the Kneipp applications (alternating warm–cold water affusions or alternating warm–cold showers), PEMF therapy, and oxygen and ozone therapies are effective.

Sports and Physical Exercise

Exercise and sports are also very important for the ABB. Depending on your fitness level, even regular walking or, if possible, light jogging at a maximum heart rate of 120 beats per minute can be very beneficial.

Similarly, cardio training can be done as a variation of endurance training at home or in a gym with the help of special equipment. To improve the oxygen–carbon dioxide exchange and by sweating out acidic metabolic products, the ABB is supported and the function of the heart–lung system is additionally improved.

Alkaline Procaine Infusions

One hundred milliliters of 8.4 percent sodium bicarbonate is mixed with between two and six milliliters of 2 percent procaine and administered as an infusion over thirty minutes.

Micronutrients

Magnesium (three hundred to four hundred milligrams per day), alkaline powder (mixtures of potassium citrate and sodium carbonate), zinc, manganese, coenzyme Q10, vitamin B complexes, and folic acid, as well as iron in the case of iron deficiency, have a balancing effect.

Liver Relief and Liver Remedies

For external and internal use, milk thistle extracts, dandelion extracts (also as a tea), alpha lipoic acid, and liver compresses with yarrow tea are suitable.

In the diet, emphasis should be placed on plant foods, alcohol should be strongly limited, nicotine should be avoided, and plenty of water should be drunk!

6.1.13 Find and Cure Chronic Infections

At the beginning of treatment, all obvious infections that show symptoms should be treated. The consequences of a silent inflammation, on the other hand, are much less obvious. They have to be determined by an examination and then treated specifically. Particularly important and delicate places where inflammation-promoting microorganisms can remain (undetected) for a long time include the following.

Root-Treated Teeth and Gums

Regular monitoring of the periodontium with X-rays is strongly recommended here. A visit to the dentist about every six months and a good dental hygienist are, in addition to the self-evident daily dental hygiene, among the important preventive measures for cancer, too. The gums should be checked regularly and especially for gum pockets and tartar (with periodontitis, the inflammation of the gums, being the most common form of periodontopathy).

Intestine and Microbiome

The microbiome examination of the intestine can provide information about intestinal inflammations, leaky gut syndrome, and endoparasites (amoebae, worms, protozoa) as well as the composition of the intestinal flora. Based on the microbiome results, a targeted symbiosis therapy with pro- and prebiotics can be planned. As a rule, this should be carried out strictly over three to four months. If there is a parasite infestation, it should be eliminated with the appropriate antibiotics. There are many anti-inflammatory medicines available for the treatment of intestinal inflammation; I would particularly like to highlight a combination of coffee charcoal, chamomile extract, and myrrh.

Precaution and Regular Examinations

Women should have their reproductive organs, especially the vagina and cervix, examined by their gynecologist during checkups.

Men should have their prostate examined (for chronic prostatitis, using PSA and manual examination of the prostate) by their general practitioner or urologist.

Frontal and Nasal Sinuses

The frontal and nasal sinuses can also be places where inflammation-promoting microorganisms can settle and trigger chronic complaints. If there are (chronic) complaints that cannot be determined more precisely by examining the inflammation values in the blood, there is also the possibility of specifically looking for possible bacteria or fungi by taking a nasal swab. If necessary, the ear, nose, and throat specialist can then select an antibiotic very specifically.

6.2 Diagnosis of Cancer: Making the Right Decisions

After a cancer diagnosis, it is important to make the right decisions: Which path should I take? The one advised to me by classical oncology, or are there other paths, alternatives?

My advice is to set out to find your own path and to look for not just one, but several specialists for the team of treating physicians or therapists. Patients should always consider this perspective: "It is my life that is at stake. I am the sovereign. I am the focus and from now on I will do only what I trust in and what feels good. I am taking my path through this crisis and doing what I believe will help me to get well again."

In Oscar Carl Simonton's seminars for sufferers, this sentiment was central, and all participants were called upon to say it out loud in front of everyone in the seminar. I remember very well how difficult this was for many, as they did not dare to claim these words for themselves. The skepticism was great, as it could also reflect their truth. Two basic beliefs often stood in their way.

1. I cannot or am not allowed to decide for myself; others must do that.
2. I cannot get better at all.

Only when these two unhealthy beliefs could be let go and replaced by healthy basic assumptions could the participants say:

"I decide to do from now on what I believe will help me to get well again!"

My advice is to write this sentence down and read it aloud again and again. There is tremendous power in it. Whether it is a difficult operation, chemotherapy or radiation, or a complementary medical treatment, none of the therapies can have their full healing effect if they are basically doubted, if they are started with fear and pessimism and ultimately only endured because others, whether doctors or family members, expect them from you.

Take your time to make the decision that is right for you, and seek as much advice and information as you need to be completely sure of what you want.

The only exceptions to this advice are emergencies in which you have to act very quickly. These can be, for example, an emergency operation to avert an immediate threat to life, a blood transfusion if the blood values have dropped to life-threatening levels, severe blood poisoning that has to be treated with antibiotics, or something similar. In most cases, however, after receiving a cancer diagnosis, you have days, often weeks, to inform yourself well and comprehensively in order to then make the right choice. Your choice!

Of course, these days or weeks should not be wasted, and the need to find a way or approach that is right for you should not be pushed to the back of your mind. The desire to bury one's head in the sand—like the proverbial ostrich—is certainly more than understandable after a shocking diagnosis, but from the day a cancer diagnosis is made, I advise you to regard it as your main task to seek immediate and comprehensive advice—as far as this is possible, but calmly and with composure—and only after receiving it to make a decision. As I've already said, I urgently warn against making a hasty decision, especially due to the attitude "I have to do what others say," or "I have to do something for others."

Among my patients, there are many who reported how they were sometimes even threatened: "If you don't start chemotherapy immediately, you'll be dead in three months." I consider this kind of "advice" to be unmedical! Don't let yourself be threatened. Incidentally, in the jargon of modern psychotherapy (for example, the school of Milton Erickson), this is called a "medical curse," which can often have disastrous effects on the health of the "cursed" person if they believe it. Examples of how to counter this can be found in section 6.1.7, "Stress Reduction: Regaining the Psychoemotional Oscillatory Capacity," page 191.

Weighing the Pros and Cons of Oncological Treatment

All oncological treatments aim to either cure or, if that is unlikely, to prolong life, reduce suffering, and improve quality of life. Most of the classic treatments of modern oncology sometimes have side effects or entail drastic changes to your life.

For the chance of being able to live longer through a treatment, it is of the upmost importance for both the treating physician and the patient to make a personal assessment: How willing is the patient to accept certain kinds of side effects and to what extent or degree? It is a central part of my daily work to consider these things together with the patient in order to reach a joint decision.

You should therefore look for a doctor who is willing to do just that with you. In my experience, many patients know too little about what expectations are realistic regarding the benefits of specific oncological treatment, and many doctors do not communicate this openly enough.

The argument that there is no time for this kind of education and engagement with the existing treatment options shows only how exaggerated the relationship is between the cost of the drugs and the resources provided in order to adequately educate patients. For example, in a three-minute conversation, therapies are recommended that cost five to six figures for a few months, while the patients are not given the chance to understand that in the worst case, no life extension at all or an average life extension of only 2.7 months (as explained in chapter 1) can be expected, sometimes with severe side effects.

A question I am often asked concerns the effect of radiation treatment for cancer. I can only advise you at this point to inform yourself precisely in this field in order to find out whether radiotherapy appears to be sensible or not. In some cases, radiotherapy of a bone metastasis, a brain tumor, or a brain metastasis may be the only thing that can quickly counteract the severe symptoms or the threat that it poses. On the other hand, in the case of an additionally recommended radiation of a certain body region, but where no visible cancerous tumors can be currently found, in order to reduce the risk of a relapse, the advantages and disadvantages should be weighed very carefully.

How Can I Draw Conclusions from Statistical Values Presented in Medical Studies?

Statistics is a complex science. It was developed as a mathematical discipline to make predictions based on observations that are believed to be relevant to the occurrence of the events being studied. If a statistical probability of an event occurring is greater than 95 percent and the probability of being wrong is less than 5 percent, we speak of a significant correlation between cause and effect.

We speak of a significant effect of a certain treatment when it can be shown within a correspondingly large study group whether the desired positive effect has occurred. If, for example, a certain form of chemotherapy or immunotherapy can measurably delay the progression of a cancer between two computed tomography (CT) examinations and the desired effect occurs 95 percent of the time, this treatment is said to have a statistically significant effect. However, this *statistically significant effect* does not yet describe how great the advantage of this treatment is.

There have been studies that attest, with statistical significance, a prolongation of life with a new type of chemotherapy, for example, in pancreatic cancer, but the actual prolongation of life was about two weeks. The relationship between the stresses and strains of this therapy and the average two weeks of life extension gained is not clear from the statement "statistically significant longer survival" alone.

You have to be trained and able to read such studies carefully to be able to classify the statement and understand the actual "advantage" described here.

If you read somewhere when searching on the internet using "Dr. Google" that there is a statistically expected average life expectancy of three years for your disease, that does not mean for you and your life that you will be dead in three years. Be very careful in assessing the literature you read about your condition and check your sources. The statistically calculated average does not have to become your reality. On average, you and the head of an international corporation are certainly billionaires, but that is usually not because of you. A statistic can illustrate what can generally be expected from a large number of studies. It cannot be a reliable prognosis or even a guarantee for events or progressions that will occur.

So if you learn something about your illness from a statistical prognosis that worries you, I hope that this "prediction" will motivate you to do more and perhaps something different from the average.

In my work as a doctor, I have met and attended to countless patients who, despite all the statistics, have lived with their disease for many years or even decades and are still alive today. They have found their path, which they trust and which has kept them alive. These patients have usually received many therapies and made changes to their lifestyle, as described in this book.

Yin and Yang: Two Different Therapeutic Principles That Complement Each Other

In Chinese philosophy and especially in Taoism, yin and yang are two polar, complementary forces that do not fight each other. I would like to use them here as an example of the two therapeutic principles of destroying cancer and supporting health or vitality. The focus of today's recognized oncology is quite clearly on the principle of destroying cancer, which is the yang principle in Taoist terms.

In classical naturopathy to orthomolecular medicine, the emphasis is placed on building up vitality and particularly on the well-functioning immune system, the supply of the mitochondria and strengthening of them, the detoxification of the organism, and much more. This principle is the yin side of the polarity.

Life needs both sides to be complete and takes place with the interplay of yin and yang. A yang-intensive chemotherapy should therefore be accompanied and complemented by a yin-active buildup and detoxification therapy in order to strengthen the best possible, life-promoting qualities. In the same way, an antibiotic therapy should be accompanied and supplemented by a probiotic therapy. Otherwise, a too yang-intensive therapy brings with it the well-known problems of immune deficiency, poisoning, and emaciation. A therapy based on only yin energy often cannot stop the aggressive cancer growth fast enough. Life-centered treatment encompasses both. This is integrative or holistic medicine. The therapies based on the yin principle of vitalization have already been discussed in detail in this book.

In the following, those cancer-killing therapies that are more subordinate to the yang principle will be presented, which can kill cancerous tumors in a targeted and relatively gentle manner.

6.3 Special Tumor-Killing Treatment Methods

Cancer-reducing or locally tumor-killing therapy methods that have few or no significant side effects in the area of general vitality are particularly favored by us, as they fit perfectly into our overall concept and cause little or hardly any damage to the rest of the organism.

6.3.1 Insulin-Potentiation Therapy

We carry out a series of IPT treatments on our patients (see chapter 5), which are most effective in the morning on an empty stomach. A session lasts between two and three hours. At the end of the IPT treatment, a small meal is served to bring the blood sugar back to normal. Depending on the severity of the condition, up to three IPT treatments are given per week for several weeks. After four to six IPT treatments and then a waiting period of about two weeks to allow the therapy to take full effect, a checkup is carried out. Depending on the clinical picture, this is done with the help of ultrasound, CT, magnetic resonance imaging (MRI), or PET-CT examinations or the determination of tumor markers in the blood. In this way, it can be assessed whether the patient has responded to the treatment, and if so, how well. The continuation of the treatment is planned on this basis.

6.3.2 Local Radio Wave Hyperthermia

We treat our patients with series of local radio wave hyperthermia (see chapter 5) up to four times a week, one hour each time. In parallel, we administer infusions with mostly biological anticancer substances. After approximately twelve such treatments, we evaluate the effect by determining tumor markers, if the tumor produces any; ultrasound, in case the tumor is visible with ultrasound; and one of the following techniques: CT, MRI, or PET-CT examination, depending on the clinical picture.

6.3.3 Photodynamic Therapy

For treatment with PDT (see chapter 5), there are a few specialized clinics in Germany, each with their own speciality. PDT can be applied several times, usually once every one to two months, and is usually not limited by side effects. It is important that the laser source is sufficiently strong and that the light-sensitive substance (photosensitizer) is well studied with regard to its absorption behavior. We work exclusively with the photosensitizer chlorin e6, which is manufactured in GMP quality by a German pharmacy. This "good manufacturing practice" is used for medicinal products for which there is a fixed set of rules.

For PDT of superficial skin tumors that do not penetrate deeper than three millimeters into the skin, but also for chronic inflammations of the skin, 5-aminolevulinic acid—an active substance from the group of photosensitizers, also called 5ALA—can be used as a cream. It leads only to the production of a photoactive substance (protoporphyrin IX) in the diseased cells, which, under the influence of the laser light, forms aggressive oxygen for seconds, which in turn causes cell death.

6.3.4 Interventional Radiology Treatments

Interventional radiology is a new speciality of radiologists who perform not only diagnostic imaging, but also special treatments: During minimally invasive procedures, special treatment catheters are inserted and combined with X-ray or CT/MRI examinations.

Metastases in the liver or lungs can be successfully treated in this way at special clinics with local chemotherapy accompanied by sclerotherapy of the blood vessels leading to the tumor, called transarterial chemoembolization (TACE). For more than fifteen years, I have been working with interventional radiologists who perform the local, minimally invasive treatment on our patients. In this procedure, a special catheter is pushed through the femoral artery into or as close as possible to the tumor under X-ray control. TACE is available for tumors from three to ten centimeters in diameter. For smaller tumors up to about three centimeters in size, for example, in the liver, another highly precise treatment method is available: sclerotherapy with radiofrequency, also called radiofrequency ablation. Both treatments are gentle on all organs that are not treated and are usually very well tolerated. My experience with both methods has been very good. We integrate them into our overall therapy concept after individual consideration in those cases in which they seem to make sense.

6.3.5 Radioligand Therapy

In certain situations, a special therapy such as radioligand therapy, which irradiates the cancer tissue from the inside, is a valuable treatment method.

It can reduce the size of the tumor in a targeted way and with relatively few side effects, or in some cases even destroy it completely. It is offered at university clinics or institutes for nuclear medicine. Examples of cases in which radioligand therapy is successfully used are metastasized prostate carcinoma and neuroendocrine tumors or carcinomas.

At the beginning of the treatment, an examination with a special PET-CT is used to check whether a certain surface receptor is present on the cancer cells of the respective patient so that the radioactive drug can bind there. If these receptors are present, the therapy can be carried out: A radioactive drug bound to a protein is injected into the vein and docks onto the cancer cell with the help of the protein. After the radioactive drug (e.g., lutetium, yttrium, or radon) has docked, the radiation, which reaches only a few centimeters, causes damage and gradual death of the tumor cells. After a few days, the radioactivity stops naturally due to the decay of the radioactive drug. The treatment usually requires three days of inpatient clinical care and is subjectively usually very well tolerated. Side effects are mainly a reduction of the hematopoietic cells in the bone marrow, which also represents the limits of the method. In difficult situations, however, it is a promising option, which we integrate into our overall concept for our patients.

6.4 Assessment Criteria, Cancer Therapies, and the Management of Cancer

6.4.1 Assessment Criteria in the Diagnosis of Oncological Diseases

After an imaging examination has been performed, the radiologist first describes what the images show and then gives an assessment. Since 2000, this has been done according to the international RECIST criteria (response evaluation criteria in solid tumors). Simplified, this means that the radiological examination result is divided into four categories:

Complete response (CR): all cancer lesions (changes caused by cancer) have disappeared.

Partial response (PR): tumor formation has decreased; the lengths of all cancer lesions have decreased by at least 30 percent.

Progressive disease (PD): progression of the disease. The sum of the longitudinal axes of the cancer lesions has increased by at least 20 percent, or new cancer lesions have formed.

Stable disease (SD): neither PR nor PD.

The first three criteria indicate that the therapy administered so far has been beneficial, as it can be assumed that the disease would have progressed without therapy. If disease progression is measured after therapy, this means that the therapy has not brought about the desired response and a new and better, more effective therapy should be found and implemented.

How Do You Evaluate Cancer Therapy?

IS THERE A "CURE" FOR CANCER?

The shortest definition of *cure* is "to live a long life." An important question here is: with how much or how little active cancer tissue? Part of living with cancer is getting regular checkups. How often one is examined and what kind of examination it is depends on many factors and is, among other things, the subject of the "guidelines" that are written and constantly improved for the different forms and stages of cancer. The current guideline on breast cancer is 390 pages long. To summarize it and all other guidelines would go beyond the scope of this book. In the following, I would like to give a brief overview of the most common examination methods and explain the terms used in therapy evaluations. This will help all those affected to carry out an evaluation of the therapy together with their doctor, from which they can make further decisions about continuing or changing the therapy. The oncological examination methods that are currently possible are as follows.

- Manual palpation of individual body regions and organs
- Ultrasound examination, which provides good images especially in areas of the body with a high fluid content, but cannot image the air-filled organs (for example, lungs and gastrointestinal tract)
- Radiological examination methods, also called imaging examination methods, such as X-ray or CT examination

- Magnetic resonance tomography (MRT; also called nuclear spin), which provides an image with very good resolution of the organs, even in the vicinity of bones
- Scintigraphy, for bones or the thyroid gland, for example
- PET-CT examination

The latter combines a metabolic analysis using a radioactive sugar molecule (PET) with a rotating X-ray camera (CT). The result is an image of the entire body and its organs, showing the degree of sugar absorption in different colors. Cancerous tissue and inflamed regions absorb ten to fifteen times more sugar than healthy tissue. PET-CT is therefore very suitable for finding metastases throughout the body.

However, none of these methods can exclude or detect cancer with certainty.

If no signs of cancer are found with an appropriate test or examination method, this is called *no evidence of disease* (NED).

However, since all diagnostic methods have a threshold below which they cannot detect minute amounts of cancer cells, tumor proteins in the blood, or tumor tissues in an imaging diagnostic, this does not mean that our organism is completely free of cancer cells or—in the case of a previous disease—is ever "cured." As already mentioned, the human organism is not completely free of cancer cells anyway, even in normal cases.

6.4.2 The Biopsy and the Significance of Tissue Examination

If the result of an examination is a "pathological finding," we first speak of a "suspicion" of a tumor disease, behind which a benign cell proliferation or a cancer disease can be hidden. Only the pathological examination of a tissue sample (biopsy), whether solid or liquid, can reliably exclude or determine a cancerous disease. No reputable doctor would forgo such a tissue examination by the pathologist before starting a treatment method specifically chosen for this type of disease.

Again and again, patients ask me how high the risk is of spreading cancer cells into the bloodstream through such a tissue removal and thus possibly paving the way for dangerous metastases. In most cases, I strongly advise patients to have a tissue examination. The exceptions to this rule of always having a biopsy done are very rare and must be decided on a case-by-case basis and with regard to special circumstances. As is so often the case in medicine, careful consideration of the advantages and possible disadvantages should be discussed with the patient in such cases. How high is the risk of having a biopsy and how high is the risk if you don't have a biopsy and thus do not receive a clear diagnosis and possibly are unable to choose the appropriate therapy because the tissue type of the tumor is not known? Modern oncology is increasingly using specific drugs whose success can be expected only in a certain form of cancer with certain biological characteristics (presence of hormone receptors, assignment of a genetic variation of a cancer form). Without a laboratory examination of the specific cell biological characteristics of a tumor tissue, these agents cannot be selected or used at all.

Only the pathological examination provides a reliable diagnosis and further important details that can help in the choice of therapy. The aim should be to be able to carry out a complete genetic analysis of the tumor tissue in order to be able to select the most effective drugs on the basis of the genetic properties of the tissue sample examined, drugs that can specifically act on that tissue.

Another problem, however, is the heterogeneity (the very often non-uniform cell types that make up a single tumor nodule) of a tumor tissue, which—the longer it has lived in the organism and has also survived anti-cancer drugs—consists of different cell clones and therefore cannot be killed by a single drug. Tumor markers can be measured in the blood for many types of cancer. These are, among other things, proteins that are also found in healthy organisms, but only in small amounts. If an organism harbors a cancer colony that produces these special proteins in larger quantities than healthy cells do, an increased value of tumor markers is found in the blood.

Cancers that have reliable tumor markers include prostate, ovarian, testicular, colon, gallbladder, pancreatic, and liver cancers.

Cancers with partially reliable tumor markers are breast, lung, uterine and cervical cancers, and neuroendocrine tumors. For at least fifteen years, there has also been talk of circulating cancer cells, also called CTCs (circulating tumor cells), in the blood. However, since there are still no reliable standards regarding the type of measurement and definition of standard values, I generally advise against relying on the purely quantitative measurement of CTCs until the measurement methods are better developed.

CTCs are also used for chemosensitivity tests, in which the effect of a drug on tumor cells is measured in the laboratory in order to predict to what extent this drug could be successfully used in the patient. As an alternative to CTCs, such a test can also be performed on a tissue sample. In discussions with cancer specialists Hans Bojar and Martin Luzbetak, I was able to understand that CTCs are very well suited for these laboratory tests. The interpretation of such a chemosensitivity test is very complex and belongs in the hands of doctors who are very familiar with it. Our experience with chemosensitivity tests is very good. They help us to optimize the choice of drugs for our treatments.

As mentioned at the beginning of this book, the state of health cannot be defined by the absence of signs of disease alone. Every medical examination therefore provides, in the best case, indications for assessing the state of health. Initially, no more and no less. The interpretation of the examination results should be carried out by a specialist, with whom patients should discuss the steps of therapy, in order to then decide what seems sensible to them and what they believe in. Healthy and ill are two (end) points on a scale, between which there can be many other things. I know people who feel ill all the time and suffer a lot, although they have no measurable, objective findings, and I know cancer patients who carry a large tumor burden and feel healthy. Which of them is really healthy?

What Can I Do If I Am Diagnosed with Cancer for the First Time?

Getting a cancer diagnosis usually comes as a shock. People who are diagnosed with cancer (for the first time) feel as if the rug is being pulled out from under their feet. Everything spins like a merry-go-round; they want to run away or feel as if they are falling into a deep hole. Some people will subsequently feel as though it doesn't affect them, as if the diagnosis is none of their business, as if they have walked into the "wrong film."

Many patients reported that they no longer heard what else the doctor said when they told them about the cancer diagnosis.

What they described afterward was a shock and a kind of trance. Some of them had a *blackout* or in extreme cases even lost consciousness for a short time, symptoms that a psychologist would call "dissociation." The consciousness, the soul, separates itself from the body for a moment. What often takes place in these first seconds is our fight-or-flight reaction, which is millions of years old and neurologically laid out in the limbic system of our brain. It expresses the deep human need to react, to be able to "do" something to change or improve the situation, and if possible, to end it.

Contrary to this natural flight or avoidance reaction, however, it is particularly important after this initial shock phase to calm down and give yourself time. Talking to your next of kin, your partner, your best friend and spending time with the people you're close to is the most important thing to do now in order to process the news of such a drastic change in your life and to be able to reorient yourself.

This can take days or even weeks. The best ways to digest the threatening news are those that provide warmth, security, and a deep sense of connection, and that may have already helped you personally before to calm down and do something good for yourself. Warming yourself up, wrapping yourself in blankets, being massaged with lavender oil—perhaps also by loved ones—or taking warm baths, going for a long run or walk, and seeking inner reflection in prayer or meditation, as well as expressing your own feelings through writing, painting, or other creative activities, are good means of being able to process the threatening news, to accept the status quo before visions can be developed.

The next step is then to become fully informed: Which treatments are available for this type of cancer? Which other examinations are important and useful? Seek advice from specialists you trust. And if your trust is not there yet or does not materialize, keep looking. In any case, seek advice and support from therapists or coaches who are experienced in psycho-oncology, counseling and support for cancer patients. Seek further advice from doctors or therapists who are well-versed in complementary medicine and can accompany you in optimizing your life forces in the sense of the twelve vital fields. However, do not expect your oncologist to devote too much time and interest to this. Very few of the oncologists I have met have any time for or interest in psycho-oncology, detoxification, or nutritional medicine. Inform your oncologist about the additional measures you are taking, but do not be put off by blanket warnings such as nutritional supplements being

unnecessary and weakening the effectiveness of chemotherapy. Unfortunately, I have frequently heard these sweeping statements without having
ever seen any substantiated evidence that the statement is true.

However, be careful with additional treatments during the intensive phases
of oncology treatment: In any case, consult an experienced doctor who can
point out possible interactions or unfavorable effects of complementary
medicine methods during oncological treatments and guide you through the
process. At the least, after an operation, chemotherapy, or radiation you have
every reason to do something to build up your intestinal flora or support
your liver detoxification.

I highly recommend that you put together a team of advisers with whom
you can master this crisis with a good conscience. In addition to the classical oncological counseling and treatment, which you (and no one else!) can
accept in part or in whole, I also recommend an experienced doctor or therapist for the areas of emotional and mental-spiritual support as well as for
the area of vital field therapy. Ideally, the complementary medicine doctor is
the link between the team members. They should provide you with so much
information that you feel safe and believe that you are taking the right path
and can always check and evaluate your progress with your team.

Preventive Examinations That Are Sensible Even without Suspicion of Cancer

For women, self-examination of the breasts is of utmost importance. Breast
cancer is the most common type of cancer in women, with over seventy
thousand new cases in Germany every year. Men are only very rarely
affected (only about 1 percent of all breast cancer patients are men, mostly
at an older age).

Once a month, preferably one week after menstruation, every woman
should examine her breasts herself. It is advisable to do this with a little
shower gel and water, for example, as this is the best way to feel for small
changes such as lumps or hardening. Every woman should therefore be well
aware of any cycle-dependent changes in her breasts so that she can detect
them herself at an early stage and have them examined by a doctor if there is
any suspicion of a lump or hardening of the breast, if the nipple has changed,
or if the skin of the breast is permanently red.

In younger men, testicular cancer is the most common type of cancer, and from around the age of fifty, it is prostate, lung, and bowel cancer.

For five types of cancer, there are currently screening programs available in Germany that can be used on your own initiative and are reimbursed by the statutory health insurance funds from a certain age, depending on the type of cancer. The cancer screening consists of examinations for the early detection of breast cancer (from the age of thirty), bowel cancer (from the age of fifty), cervical cancer (from the age of thirty-five), skin cancer (from the age of thirty-five), and prostate cancer (from the age of forty-five). They can be carried out by general practitioners or specialists.

In addition, there is a supplementary diagnosis method called thermography of the female breast, which produces a thermal image of the body surface without any side effects. For this method, thermal images of the breasts are taken first before and then again after fifteen minutes of cooling at a room temperature of about 21°C (70°F) and with the upper body undressed. Regions of the breast where there is either inflammation or tumor growth are usually overheated and cool down less quickly than healthy areas. Although there is already a lot of knowledge about breast thermography, unfortunately this method is still not promoted enough by larger clinical studies or offered to patients in oncological centers; there is a lack of lobbying. In my practice, it has been an important additional method for monitoring female breast health for a good ten years and, compared to classical X-ray mammography, it is completely free of side effects.

As a general rule, bleeding from the intestines or colon should always be clarified by a doctor. It can be harmless in nature (for example, caused by tears in the anal mucosa or hemorrhoids), but it can also be a sign of colorectal or intestinal cancer. In general, the risk of cancer increases with age. Older people, and this also applies to "young-at-heart" people in their sixties, should therefore have their health checked regularly.

6.5 The Treatment of Leukemia: A "Liquid" Form of Cancer

Until about seventy years ago, a diagnosis of acute leukemia was tantamount to a death sentence. No treatment could stop its rapid and invariably fatal progression, until 1947, when the American pathologist Sidney Farber first used a cell poison that counteracted folic acid and killed the immature leukemia cells. Although the treatment was initially successful only in prolonging life by a few months, it ushered in the age of chemotherapy, which has since been further refined and intensively researched.

Today, leukemia patients have a comparatively good prognosis, depending on the type and stage. Therefore, they should definitely turn to a treatment center that has a lot of experience with this. These are usually university hospitals. In my entire professional career, I have not come across any effective alternative to them. In the case of leukemia, the task of complementary medicine is to provide support through the "terrain therapies," as illustrated in this book using the example of the twelve vital fields, as support before and after the special hemato-oncological treatment in a university hospital.

6.6 Treatment with Nononcological Drugs

In the history of pharmacology—especially that of the last century—we find many examples of only gradually discovered and additional effects of drugs that were originally developed for a different clinical picture.

The fever-reducing painkiller acetylsalicylic acid (ASA), for example, also known as aspirin, only acquired its additional significance as a blood-thinning drug in the prophylactic care of strokes or heart attacks many decades after it was introduced.

The development of the blood-sugar-lowering type 2 diabetes drug metformin was similar; it has been known for some years to reduce the risk of cancer or slow its growth. In January 2020, a study was published in the renowned journal *Nature* describing how 4,518 drugs were tested for their growth-inhibiting properties in laboratory experiments on 518 different human cancer cell lines from a total of 24 different types of cancer. In the process, 49 nononcological drugs were found, each of which showed a killing effect of cancer cells in a weaker or stronger form. The publication concluded that these drugs, which have shown to be effective in clinical use, should be investigated in further clinical trials to ensure safe use. However, the problem with funding such studies is that the patents for many of these drugs have already expired and thus the economic motivation is lacking, since no (additional) money can be earned with them. But this is not a satisfactory perspective for those who are suffering from cancer today and are looking for means to prolong their lives while maintaining their quality of life. After all, there is a growing number of patients who use these drugs for themselves, and doctors who want to help them.

English physiotherapist, author, and cancer survivor Jane McLelland described in her biography how she recovered from stage four metastatic cervical cancer. At the end of the book, she described in detail what she has studied for years and ultimately applied to herself: the nononcological drugs (also known as repurposed drugs or off-label drugs), which stopped her cancer growth and thereby restored the inner balance between healthy and diseased cells. McLelland described three metabolic pathways of cancer in particular, which can be blocked with drugs originally developed for other diseases. This prevents the vital energy supply for the cancer cells, which in the best case starves them out. The drugs she mentioned are the type 2 diabetes drug metformin, mentioned above, and dipyridamole (an anti-inflammatory, thrombosis-preventing drug mainly used to prevent strokes), mebendazole (a drug against worm infestation), atorvastatin (a drug to lower blood fat levels), and doxycycline, a classic antibiotic.

During two personal encounters with Jane McLelland at conferences in England in 2018 and in the United States in 2019, I was able to get a firsthand impression of her vitality and enthusiasm for her discoveries as she presented parts of her book. While her formula can provide many suggestions for doctors and sufferers, there is once again no single panacea for successful treatment of cancer. Since I first became acquainted with it, her book has been a constant stimulus for me to look for other non- or only slightly debilitating methods and remedies with which my patients can further control their cancers.

What all drugs not approved for cancer treatment have in common is that they have relatively minor or less aggressive side effects compared to the classical chemotherapy drugs. They can all be taken in the dose individually determined by a doctor, even in the long term, and cost comparatively little. Another common characteristic is that they each inhibit one of the three most important metabolic pathways of cancer cells: They either impair the supply of glucose, affect amino acids/glutamine, or reduce the fat metabolism of cancer cells. In recent years, a practical place to go for prescribing off-label drugs for cancer has been the London Care Oncology Clinic. Some of our patients have been able to get prescriptions there, mainly for the four drugs mentioned above, to help them curb their cancer: the type 2 diabetes drug metformin, the blood-lipid-lowering drug atorvastatin, the anti-parasite drug mebendazole, and the antibiotic doxycycline. Doctors experienced in the use of these drugs decide which drugs can be taken and in which dosage regimen, depending on the type of tumor. After regular evaluation of the course of the disease, the intake protocol is either maintained or changed if necessary, depending on the success.

Other examples of off-label use for cancer are sildenafil, better known as Viagra, for which there are indications of positive effects in colorectal cancer; beta-blockers (especially in ovarian cancer); the drug disulfiram, which is actually used for relapse prophylaxis in alcoholism; the anti-inflammatory celecoxib, which is used, for example, for joint inflammation; and the tried and tested painkiller and addiction substitute methadone.

The chemist Claudia Friesen, who conducts research at the university hospital in Ulm, Germany, discovered as early as 2008 that methadone (especially a mixture of two different forms of methadone: D,L-methadone) had a specific effect on cancer cells in laboratory experiments, which, among other things, inhibited their cellular detoxification. With her publications from 2008 to 2014, which were later also discussed in media such as daily newspapers, radio programs, and television programs, she triggered not only great hope but also a veritable storm of criticism. Doctors who prescribe D,L-methadone as a painkiller for their pain-stricken tumor patients have been able to see for years that it not only helps to control the pain caused by the tumor well and with few side effects, but also has a synergistic effect with other cancer-killing therapies. Of course, further clinical studies on this would be more than desirable. However, the same problem as just described is that because this is a very inexpensive drug and therefore produces little profit for its makers (it was already developed and used in World War II as a painkiller with a mood-lifting effect), further studies can never be financed: "Life has its price: methadone could possibly help thousands of cancer patients. Yet the substance is not being researched because it promises too little profit."[9]

I would like to expressly warn against experimenting with these remedies yourself without involving an experienced doctor. The drugs mentioned here all require a prescription and have side effects that need to be weighed against the risks of a progressive cancer by an experienced doctor or therapist. They may interact with other medicines and should always be monitored by a doctor for the duration of use.

6.7 From the "Point of No Return" and Palliative Care

In many cases and often after many years of intensive therapies, cancer leads to a point at which the progression of the disease can no longer be stopped. Apart from courses of the illness bordering on miracles, of which there are some documented cases, many people have to come to terms with this fact again and again. This is also a difficult situation for doctors and therapists. If the tumor burden on the one hand and the weakening of the vital field on the other hand is too great, after a certain point medical treatments can often no longer do anything against the advancement of the tumor spread. Certain treatment methods may still be available, but from a certain point they are no longer fast and effective enough. The relationship between side effects and the desired anticancer effect shifts more and more toward side effects after a certain point. It then sometimes seems like a Sisyphean task. This acknowledgment is an incredibly difficult but also important insight that needs to be discussed with patients and their relatives.

Several times in my life as a doctor I have met patients who told me just a few days before or even on the day of their death that they never wanted to give up and now felt that their healing was close. Only with a spiritual understanding of life and death can one guess what these people felt or recognized, and what the German poet Novalis described in a poem:

> In everlasting life death found its goal,
> For thou art Death who at last makes us whole.

Understanding and accepting this conditionality and preparing patients to die is an important task for the doctor, which is often accompanied by very ambivalent feelings of powerlessness. Addressing death as inevitable and also preparing the relatives to talk to the dying person about death and their fears, beliefs, or wishes in the case of death is an important therapeutic measure in the last stage of cancer treatment.

In any case, supportive medical treatment can and should be available until the end in order to alleviate pain, nausea, and fears and to maintain the quality of life as far as possible. Doctors also refer to this as *best supportive care*, whereby the supportive therapies can also merge into palliative medical care.

The word *palliative* (from the Latin *palliare*) actually means "to wrap with a cloak" and is a treatment that alleviates the discomfort of an illness but can no longer combat its causes. Thinking palliatively means continuing to support life and accepting death as a natural process. Palliative medicine in the narrower sense means maintaining the highest possible quality of life in a life situation in which there can no longer be an effective treatment for cancer, where tumor reduction is not possible. From this point on, it is no longer a matter of giving life more days, but of giving the days more life. However, the word *palliative* is often used in a completely different way, for example, when oncologists assume that there is no longer any prospect of a complete response to treatment. Palliative medicine and palliative treatments can, however, sometimes last for many years.

It is a blessing that modern drug therapy provides us with effective and safe means that can also cope with the severe symptoms and pain of the last days and enable a dignified end of life. Conversation and human closeness are not only important here, but are indispensable.

6.8 Inner Life Training

6.8.1 Realigning Body, Mind, and Spirit with the Power of Positive Affirmations

Adaptability is the highly successful survival strategy used throughout nature. From the life of bacteria to cells to the highly complex human being, life finds a way to overcome challenges, survive and persevere, and thrive by being adaptable. Adaptability means adjusting one's behavior according to circumstances. "When life gives you lemons, make lemonade" humorously expresses this concept. How *healing* is to be understood and what dynamic process this word should actually describe has already been explained in this book in various contexts. Our organism is never completely free of disease-producing factors. But how we deal with this fact and which parts of ourselves we want to strengthen is the decisive key to a healthier, more contented life. The knowledge that, due to our evolutionary development, we do not have only one brain in the form of a single "being" that influences and directs our behavior can help here. We have at least three areas in our brain that work together more or less efficiently. In addition, there are other *subpersonalities* or *ego states* that contribute to what we call our "personality." Depending on the quality of what we experience, one part or another of our brain is activated and dominates our behavior. As already mentioned with regard to the limbic stress response (page 121), there are different parts of our brain that evolution has formed:

- The conscious part, which is mainly located in the frontal lobe
- The midbrain, which comprises the limbic system and the amygdala
- The brainstem, where the archaic and basic instincts or behavior patterns are located

Changes should therefore take place not only in our daily lives (for example, through behavioral changes or dietary changes), but also in our minds, so that we can adapt optimally, react adequately, when cancer becomes a fact in our lives. If we are directly affected, the cancer condition or any other life-threatening disease we live with triggers a high level of uncertainty and fear and the fight-or-flight reflex, described above, in our brain. So this is where our primeval heritage comes into play, and we must decide in a flash whether it makes sense to flee or fight. The "switch" or the center of this stress reaction is the *amygdala* (from ancient Greek and also described as an almond-shaped nucleus). It is located in the midbrain and is part of the limbic system, which is also called the "reptilian brain" because of its early developmental history. This *alarm center* causes a lot of emotional discomfort when it comes to life-threatening news. Emotions ranging from mild fear to great panic are caused, among other things, by the release of stress hormones, and it is these same stress and fear reactions that block the immune system and many important self-healing functions, but which are switched on as soon as we understand that our lives are at stake. They are emergency reactions designed to get us out of a dangerous situation within seconds or minutes. So the amygdala is not designed to "befriend" an enemy or find a way to cope with cancer. This is another reason why the term *reptilian brain* fits quite well. The release of stress hormones such as cortisol, adrenaline, and noradrenaline generates immediate energy for fight or flight, as if cancer were a predator threatening our lives with an attack at this very second. But if the life-threatening challenge is not a wild beast or an aggressive warrior, this ancient fight-or-flight reaction is the wrong response to stress.

Another, third stress response that has survived evolutionary development is *freezing*. When our ancestors could not escape the saber-toothed tiger (the archetypal aggressor of earlier times) because it was already too close and both flight and fight seemed hopeless, they played dead, they froze. These were good strategies a few thousand years ago, when danger in life came from wild animals, war, or aggressive neighbors. But they are actually bad strategies when the danger is a chronic disease. But this is how we can understand why we feel powerless, numb, paralyzed, or depressed and "freeze" in response to some situations; but also why we scream, run, choose harmful therapies, and need to do something, immediately, here and now (fight), or why we deny and refuse to acknowledge certain things like a cancer diagnosis (flight).

The old reason our amygdala is programmed to feel safe is to eliminate the predator. In the case of metastatic cancer, however, this program does not help. It makes us fearful and weak in the long run. It does us no favors. In fact, it can even ruin our lives.

As advanced as humanity may feel in parts, in this case, evolution—equipped with the genes and behavioral patterns of our ancestors—has not prepared us well enough to deal optimally with long-term life-threatening challenges. Therefore, we must learn a new strategy! The intelligent brain, located in the frontal lobe behind the forehead, can learn a better way: controlling cancer cells through your immune system and your self-healing powers. So if the amygdala functions like a "smoke detector" that protects us from possible "fire hazards" and warns us as soon as there is "smoke" in the air, we need to recalibrate it if we live near "open fire" or a "smoky" area—in other words, if cancer is a part of the body and of life.

We need to find a *new normal* and accept the fact that cancer cells are present. The uncertainty that comes with it must be accepted by our *danger detector* and become part of the "new" normal life that will never be the same again. The sooner we accept it, the better we will cope with our condition, prognosis, and life.

This recalibration will take time and requires practice in the brain and psyche. We need to learn the language that the amygdala speaks and understands. Clinical hypnosis uses communication techniques that bridge the path from consciousness to the subconscious limbic system where the amygdala operates. One of these techniques, for example, is inner life training (ILT), as presented below. The healing meditations listed below also work according to the same principle.

After more than twenty-five years of practical experience, I can assure you that this is an essential part of the changes to live longer and better, no matter what stage of your cancer condition you are in. Using knowledge of how stress patterns work to learn an optimal strategy for coping with cancer will make your life more enjoyable, reduce anxiety and stress, and give you a longer and better quality of life. Your subconscious will slowly and surely allow the new normal and reduce the stress signals each time you practice ILT. After a period of practice, the *new normal* will become a new and healthy attitude and give you the best mental prerequisite for improving your health.

6.8.2 How to Practice Inner Life Training

Sit comfortably on a chair. Your upper body is erect. Legs and arms are not crossed but parallel and—if you wish—your palms are facing upward and resting on your thighs. If it feels better and *more grounded* for you to stand, your feet should be hip-width apart, with your knees as far apart as possible and your arms hanging loosely at your sides.

Feel the floor under your feet, feel the weight of your body resting on the chair. Feel your breath. Breathe a little deeper and slower.

Use your abdominal muscles to breathe. Feel your abdomen protruding as you breathe in and contracting as you breathe out. Try to keep your shoulders relaxed. Breathe with only your abdomen. Breathe slowly.

You can slow down your breathing by exhaling with slight resistance created by your lips or by exhaling through one nostril only and holding the other nostril closed with your index finger (a technique used in yoga).

Slow breathing is a very effective way of switching off the production of stress hormones within a few minutes and stimulating your parasympathetic nervous system, that part of your autonomic nervous system that represents self-healing, regeneration, good digestion, muscle relaxation, and good feelings. After a few minutes of conscious, slow breathing, you can focus on an affirmation that you like to practice. Affirmations are inner words or thoughts that create good feelings, give hope, and are based on truth and compassion. Affirmations work most powerfully when we focus on them and slowly say them to ourselves over and over again, giving the words a special color or imagined light energy, and combining them with a physical (somatic) sensation, such as gentle touch (see figure 8 in the color insert). You can also use the following formulations to practice ILT or tune into the healing meditations. Again, feel free to sit or stand, as works best for you.

- I feel my body resting safely on this chair (which is standing safely).
- I feel my breath and enjoy breathing deeply and slowly. I feel how it helps my body to heal.
- I allow myself to feel good now and let go of all the tension, the fear, the worries I had in the past. I breathe out the past and breathe in the now!
- I feel the power of life in my heart.
- I am grateful for the gift of life that moves my heart at this moment.
- I choose now to focus on the power of life that I feel in my heart and that flows from my heart into my whole body.

Gently place your hand on your heart.
- I feel the warmth of my palm and the movements of my heart, which is the center of life in my body.
- I focus on this power that I feel deep within myself, give it my favorite healing color, and let it flow through my whole body.

- Together with my breath, I feel the power of self-healing, the power in my immune system in my blood, which I let become strong again and which helps me to take good care of my health, my body, and myself.
- I have strong reasons to live my life.

6.8.3 Inner Life Training Affirmations for Both Physical and Emotional Pain

Carry out the following steps.

- Feel the pain and find out what it is. Where in your body do you feel it? What emotions are associated with the pain? Describe them.
- Focus on this point in your body where you feel the pain the most. Dare to feel it really intensely. Go to this place in your body where you feel it intensely and then do the ILT confirmation exercise from page 227. Breathe through the place in your body where you feel the pain most intensely. Feel and see with your inner eye how this spot becomes softer and softer, lighter and lighter, the more you breathe through it.
- Transform this spot in your inner imagination, and give it a meaning or a name. You can call it your healing point, which reminds you to do the ILT exercises from time to time. Thank it.
- Do not use judgmental expressions when you do affirmations. Use terms that describe acceptance or even gratitude in your statements, and avoid judgments by all means.

6.9 Healing Meditations

In section 3.8.3, "Healing Meditations: Aligning Consciousness and Promoting Coherence," page 123, we have already presented the connection between body and soul (physis and psyche) and referred to the healing meditations presented here. You can carry them out exactly as described, but they can also serve as examples to inspire your own sentences and formulations (see figure 9 in the color insert). To perform the healing meditations, sit upright and comfortably as described above or stand in a stable position before you begin.

Healing Meditation 1:
Feeling Safe in Being at One with Yourself

I feel safe in my body.
A feeling of safety flows through all my limbs with my breath.
I feel warmth in my breast, which I draw strength from.

I feel my life in my heart.
My life flows in my blood within me,
from my heart to my fingertips
and from my toes back to the center of my heart.
Everything in me is flowed through and enlivened by my blood.

In my clear consciousness, now, in this moment,
I experience my true being:
my origin, my being in the now, and my future.
It is I who contemplates them, guides them, and seizes them,
at all times.
I am timeless, always at one with myself,
I am who I am.

In the safety of my warm breast,
in the vibrant current of my blood
and my self-healing powers,
in the meaningful light of my clear consciousness,
I feel with gratitude the healing power of transformation,
how it flows through me and warms me,
and how the feeling of safety carries me through all my existence.

Healing Meditation 2:
Healing through Warmth, Life, and Light

Warmth—in my breast.

Life—in my heart.

Light—in my consciousness.

Warmth, light, and life,
they flow within me,
in healing waves,
in the rise and fall of my breath,
in the pulsing of my heart.

They weave my life force field,
they have a healing effect
in my whole body.

I feel them.

I strengthen their flow
through my breath.

I accompany them
with my inner light
in loving recognition.

I am grateful for the healing
in this moment,
in my whole life.

Healing Meditation 3: Love

The shame, there it is.
I let it go.
It slips away from me.

The guilt, I feel it.
I let it go and feel it moving on,
like a cloud in the sky.

The fear, I know it well.
I listen to it for a little while longer
and release it, calmly and safely.

The pride, I know it.
I smile at it and leave it be,
while internally I go on, to myself.

The courage, I feel it
and breathe it in.

The willingness, I feel it
and open myself up to it and my life.

The acknowledgment of what is.
I feel how much good it does me,
and look at things
and see them as they are.

Love. I am of it and in it.
I love my life and my life loves me.

I love.

Healing Meditation 4:
Meditating with the Seven Chakras

This meditation is based on the system of the seven life centers, the chakras of Tantric Buddhism (see figure 10 in the color insert). They consist of:

- the root chakra (Muladhara Chakra)
- the sacral chakra (Svadhistana Chakra)
- the solar plexus chakra (Manipura Chakra)
- the heart chakra (Anahata Chakra)
- the throat chakra (Vishudda Chakra)
- the brow chakra (Ajna Chakra, also known as the third eye)
- the crown chakra (Sahasrara Chakra)

These all lie on a straight line in the body's vertical axis. The numbers of the individual sentences stand for the respective chakra, which are assigned the numbers one to seven, starting from the bottom of the body (the root chakra in the genital area) up to the crown of the head (the crown chakra).

1. I feel the security and stability as a source of strength deep down in my pelvis, which connects me as if through a root with the life forces of Mother Earth. (genital area)
2. I feel my creativity and my creative power in my middle pelvis and let them flow freely as an expression of my femininity/ masculinity. (two fingers' width below the navel)
3. I feel my inner wisdom in my solar plexus, the willpower in the intuition of my gut feeling. (solar plexus)
4. I feel warmth and compassion in my heart. I am loved and I love. (height of the heart)

5. I feel free to express myself in the way that suits me and I communicate openly with those around me. (height of the larynx)
6. I feel my intuition and recognize myself and the world. (two fingers' width above the root of the nose, third eye)
7. I am connected with my higher self, with universal consciousness, with God. (top of the skull, highest point of the head with upright head posture)

Healing Meditation 5: The Light Meditation

In this meditation, the focus is on harmonizing our own paternal (male) and maternal (female) parts—beyond the experiences that sometimes make life difficult for us (figure 11 in the color insert). Here we can connect, in gratitude and with the help of our consciousness, with the general forces of the parental origin and, if necessary or beneficial, also in the vein of reconciliation.

In mythological terms, this meditation leads us to the original forces of Gaia (from Greek mythology, this means Mother Earth) and Uranos (who represents Heaven or Father of the Cosmos in Greek mythology). With these two forces, below and above are also represented as the conditional principle:

I feel the warming connection to the earth beneath me.

Like red warm light it flows inside me through my pelvis upward along my spine.

With each breath in, I draw this warming, security-giving, red maternal power into me and guide it with my consciousness along my spine up to my head.

I feel the clear, ordering power of the sky above me and guide it into me with my breath through my vertex along my spine.

Like a blue light, it flows into me in an ordering manner as a fatherly force.

In my heart, the red and blue waves of light unite (when inhaling) to form a violet glow, which (when exhaling) radiates from my heart shining in all directions.

I am wanted and loved by Mother and Father, and I live my life in freedom.

Cancer and a Good Life Are Not Mutually Exclusive

It may seem like a paradox at first. Receiving a cancer diagnosis can be the worst news I've had in my life, and at the same time it can be a key healing moment for a more conscious life that suits me more than the one before the diagnosis. Having cancer inside you and living a good, fulfilled life are not mutually exclusive.

How Is That Possible?

Resolving the paradox requires a differentiated view on several levels. A paradox always points to a change of level, which is necessary to resolve it. To do this, it is helpful that I pause for a moment, put aside my usual strategies of judgment, and concentrate entirely on observing what is happening. I recommend this exercise from mindfulness training to anyone interested in a deeper understanding of illness and life. An inner attitude of wonder and alert interest helps me to direct my gaze to deeper layers. What is being expressed right now in what I have experienced, what I am experiencing?

Let us imagine: A person feels a pain in his chest. He goes to the doctor, who, after examining him, tells him that the cause of the pain is a cancerous tumor that has formed. "You have cancer!" Most people are floored when they first hear this, and a state of shock ensues, often for days or weeks. Fear and the nearness of death are right in front of you and pull you in. Only a conscious inner attitude can stop this "film" and let the power flow into a path of healing.

An insight can come: Something in me has withdrawn from the healthy balance of my body. What can I do to regain this balance and to continue to live my life well, perhaps even better, to shape it and also to fill it with meaning and enjoy it again?

The philosophically profound physics Nobel Prize–winner Niels Bohr (1885–1962) once wrote the following insight in an essay: "The opposite of a correct assertion is a false assertion. The opposite of a profound truth may very well be another profound truth."

This is a paradox. The level change is expressed by the word *profound*. Cancer is a *profound* issue. A profound issue points to a profound truth. In the same way, our life and biography is a profound issue with profound truths that reveal themselves to us only gradually and through an approach requiring patience and self-knowledge.

On the physiological level, cancer is a potentially fatal disease that I want to remove from my body so as not to die too soon. On the evolutionary biological level, cancer is a regression of the development of my body's cells to a state that heralds the death of my hitherto serving, highly differentiated body. On the psychological level, cancer confronts me with suffering and with existential questions about how I have lived my life so far and how I want to live it in the future. And on the cognitive level, cancer is a constant reminder of the equilibrium nature of health on which I want to build my fulfilling life (see figure 12 in the color insert). The possibility of getting cancer is deeply woven into the life of our body's cells. Each of our cells carries with it proto-oncogenic— dormant and, when activated, cancer-triggering DNA segments—which I either prevent, throughout my life, from being implemented to produce cancer cells by living a healthy lifestyle, or activate by doing the opposite, by the gradual influence of cancer-triggering factors and the waning of health.

If I end my life at the age of one hundred with a cancerous tumor inside me, that is not a disease in the sense of this book. In this case, cancer is a natural consequence of aging and a door through which I can leave life and discard my worn-out body like an old garment. If cancer is the cause of suffering and shortening of life before I have lived my life to the full, then it is a tragic disease that needs to be alleviated or cured.

Dying with cancer after having lived my life to the fullest is no longer a misfortune. To die of cancer before I have lived my life, that is the tragedy for which this book offers a multilayered solution, but without offering a cheap promise of a cure.

The subject of this book is that, in addition to modern oncological treatments aimed at cancer elimination, there is a way to make peace with cancer, to experience it as an awakening turning point, and to decide to want to get well, regardless of the length of the healing journey, and to be prepared to live a successful life with it before it has succeeded.

Acknowledgments

Anyone who has the good fortune to write a book like this may turn with gratitude to all the people who were involved in its genesis. Without them, this book would never have come into being, and so I would like to express my gratitude here for their help and the inspiration they gave me.

First and foremost, I would like to thank my parents, who gave me the opportunity to experience a wide-ranging school education and eventually study medicine. Both of them passed away as a result of cancer. Without the important experience of witnessing as a medical student how helpless university medicine was in the face of my mother's metastasized breast cancer, my life certainly would have been very different and this book would not have been written. Twenty years later, I was then able to use a small part of what is described in this book to support my father, who was suffering from cancer and whose course of the illness over a good eleven years was much better than was feared at the beginning of his illness. In both cases, I am grateful for the life-shaping experience of supporting my parents, who were affected by cancer.

I would like to thank my teachers at the Freie Waldorfschule in Ulm for never tiring of answering my many questions in an interesting way and spurring me on to keep asking new questions. In particular, I would like to thank Helmut Neuffer, Joachim Kratzer, Dr. Henrik Weidemann, Walter Schweizer, and Reinhard Schwenk for teaching me how to observe, how to let phenomena affect and speak to me, how to marvel, and how to research.

My thanks go to my academic teachers at the University of Ulm for introducing me to the world of natural science, in particular my doctoral supervisor Dr. Roderich Hohage and the outstanding human geneticist and anthropologist Prof. Dr. Helmut Baitsch.

For the introduction into the world of psycho-oncology, I would like to thank Dr. Oscar Carl Simonton, probably the best-known pioneer in this field, whose work I'd already read as a student and who was my teacher from 2000 until his death in 2009.

I would also like to thank Ulrike Plaßmann, whose illustrations for this book opened up another congenial approach to the topics dealt with and who, moreover, tried to help me square the circle with this book. Its content had to show the scientific basics and at the same time be understandable and stimulating for everyone. Therefore, many academic concepts also had to be put into expressive pictures and words that could be generally understood.

Thank you to Chelsea Green Publishing's Margo Baldwin and Brianne Goodspeed for the practical implementation and publication of this work.

But I would also like to express my particular appreciation of you, dear reader. I thank you for your openness, your interest, and your willingness to take time for the book and to let yourself be touched by its contents.

The greatest thanks, however, go to all my patients, who have been and still are my most important teachers since I started practicing medicine.

Notes

1. *Corpus Hippocraticum*, 11.328
2. Johann Wolfgang von Goethe, "Zahme Xenien" [Tame xenias], in *Poetische Werke* [Poetic works], vol. 1, *Gedichte: Ausgabe letzter Hand 1827* [Poems: Final hand edition] (Berlin: Aufbau Verlag, 1960), 635–37.
3. Johann Wolfgang von Goethe, "Buch des Sängers" [Book of the singer], in *Poetische Werke* [Poetic works], vol. 3, *Gedichte: West-östlicher Diwan* [Poems: West-east divan] (Berlin: Aufbau Verlag, 1960), 7–9.
4. *Tao Te King* [Tao te ching], 4th ed. (DTC Klassik, 1991), verse 2.
5. Matthew 6:34 (Luther Version).
6. Gary Bruno Schmid, *Selbstheilung durch Vorstellungskraft* [Self-healing by imagination] (Heidelberg: Springer Verlag, 2011).
7. Johann Wolfgang von Goethe, "Eins und Alles" [One and all], in *Gedichte und Epen* [Poems and epics], bk. 1 (Munich: Deutscher Taschenbuch Verlag, 1998); translated into English by the author.
8. *Corpus Hippocraticum*, 1.
9. Anette Dowideit, "Leben hat seinen preis" [Life has its price], *Die Welt am Sonntag*, November 13, 2016, https://www.mamazone.de/fileadmin/downloads/Aktuelles/2016/artikel_welt_am_sonntag_friesen.pdf.

References

Introduction

Zadeh, Lofti. "Fuzzy Languages and Their Relation to Human and Machine Intelligence." *Man and Computer* (1972): 130–65. https://doi.org/10.1159/000393834. Cited in Gaines, "Foundations of Fuzzy Reasoning." *International Journal of Man-Machine Studies* 8, no. 6 (November 1976): 624. https://doi.org/10.1016/S0020-7373(76)80027-2.

Chapter 1. Who Suffers from Cancer and Who Profits from This Suffering

Der Krebsinformationsdienst des Deutschen Krebsforschungszentrums [Information service of the German cancer research center]. Accessed 2021. https://www.krebsinformationsdienst.de.

Flashar, Hellmut. *Hippokrates. Meister der Heilkunst* [Hippocrates: Master of medicine]. Munich: CH Beck Verlag, 2016.

Gøtzsche, Peter C. *Tödliche Medizin und organisierte Kriminalität. Wie die Pharmaindustrie unser Gesundheitswesen korrumpiert* [Deadly medicine and organized crime: How the pharmaceutical industry corrupts healthcare]. Munich: Riva Verlag, 2014.

Heinzerling, Lucie, Enrico N. de Toni, Georg Schett, Gheorghe Hundorfean, and Lisa Zimmer. "Checkpoint-Inhibitoren. Diagnostik und Therapie von Nebenwirkungen" [Checkpoint inhibitors: The diagnosis and treatment of side effects]. *Deutsches Ärzteblatt International* 116, no. 8 (2019): 119–26. https://doi.org/10.3238/arztebl.2019.0119.

Kleiner, P., and U. Jaehde. "Checkpointinhibitoren: Dosisindividualisierung als Schlüssel zur Kostensenkung?" [Checkpoint inhibitors: Dose individualization as key to cost reduction?] *Best Practice Onkologie* 15 (April 2020): 198–203. https://doi.org/10.1007/s11654-020-00219-2.

Swanton, Charles. "Cancer Therapeutics through an Evolutionary Lens." *Journal of the Royal Society of Medicine* 111, no. 1 (January 2018): 8–14. https://doi.org/10.1177/0141076817742096.

Tirrell, Meg. "The World Spent This Much on Cancer Drugs Last Year." *CNBC*, June 2, 2016. https://www.cnbc.com/2016/06/02/the-worlds-2015-cancer-drug-bill-107-billion-dollars.html.

Venugopal, Jisha, and Chaitanya Nandan. *What's Now and Next in Immuno-Oncology?* New York: SG Analytics Pharma and Life Sciences, 2017. https://2wpb9mpgou83870m43d4f7bp-wpengine.netdna-ssl.com/wp-content/uploads/2018/03/immuno-oncology-insights-paper.pdf. (This paper has information on the profit margins of medicines.)

World Health Organization. "Cancer Today." International Agency for Research on Cancer. Accessed 2021. https://gco.iarc.fr/today/home.

Chapter 2. How the Light Shines

Bischof, Marco. *Biophotonen. Das Licht in unseren Zellen* [Biophotons: The light in our cells]. Frankfurt: Zweitausendeins Verlag, 1995.

Braden, Gregg. *Im Einklang mit der göttlichen Matrix. Wie wir mit Allem verbunden sind* [In harmony with the divine matrix: How we are connected to everything]. Dorfen: Koha Verlag, 2007.

Endo, Hiroko, and Mashiro Inoue. "Dormancy in Cancer." *Cancer Science* 110, no. 2 (2019): 474–80. https://doi.org/10.1111/cas.13917.

Nagl, W., and F. A. Popp. "A Physical (Electromagnetic) Model of Differentiation. 1. Basic Considerations." *Cytobios* 37, no. 145 (1983): 45–62. https://pubmed.ncbi.nlm.nih.gov/6851665/.

Popp, Fritz-Albert. *Biophotonen. Neue Horizonte in der Medizin. Von den Grundlagen zur Biophotonik* [Biophotons—new horizons in medicine: From the basics to biophotonics]. Stuttgart: Haug Verlag, 2006.

Popp, F. A., and W. Nagl. "A Physical (Electromagnetic) Model of Differentiation. 2. Applications and Examples." *Cytobios* 37, no. 146 (1983): 71–83. https://pubmed.ncbi.nlm.nih.gov/6617259/.

Van Wijk, Roeland. *Light in Shaping Life: Biophotons in Biology and Medicine*. Geldermalsen: Meluna Research, 2014.

Van Wijk, R., and J. M. van Aken. "Photon Emission in Tumor Biology." *Experientia* 48 (December 1992): 1092–102. https://doi.org/10.1007/BF01947996.

Chapter 3. The Holistic Model of the Twelve Vital Fields

Drevs, Joachim. *Integrative Onkologie. Definition, Inhalte, Bedeutung* [Integrative oncology: Definition, contents, significance]. Berlin: De Gruyter Verlag, 2020.

3.1 The Detoxification of the Organism

Arauz, Jonathan, Natanael Zarco, José Segovia, Mineko Shibayama, Victor Tsutsumi, and Pablo Muriel. "Caffeine Prevents Experimental Liver Fibrosis by Blocking the Expression of TGF-β." *European Journal of Gastroenterology and Hepatology* 26, no. 2 (February 2014): 164–73. https://doi.org/10.1097/MEG.0b013e3283644e26.

Birerdinc, A., M. Stepanova, L. Pawloski, and Z. M. Younossi. "Caffeine Is Protective in Patients with Non-alcoholic Fatty Liver Disease." *Alimentary Pharmacology Therapeutics* 35, no. 1 (January 2012): 76–82. https://doi.org/10.1111/j.1365-2036.2011.04916.x.

Chen, Shaohua, Narci C. Teoh, Shiv Chitturi, and Geoffrey C. Farrell. "Coffee and Non-alcoholic Fatty Liver Disease: Brewing Evidence for Hepatoprotection?" *Journal of Gastroenterology and Hepatology* 29, no. 3 (March 2014): 435–41. https://doi.org/10.1111/jgh.12422.

Costentin, Charlotte E., Françoise Roudot-Thoraval, Elie-Serge Zafrani, Fatiha Medkour, Jean-Michel Pawlotsky, Ariane Mallat, and Christophe Hézode. "Association of Caffeine Intake and Histological Features of Chronic Hepatitis C." *Journal of Hepatology* 54, no. 6 (June 2011): 1123–29. https://doi.org/10.1016/j.jhep.2010.08.027.

Deutsches Grünes Kreuz e.V. Informationsportal für Gesundheit [German Green Cross: Information portal for health.] "Thema: Lebererkrankungen" [Theme: Liver diseases]. Accessed 2021. https://www.kaffee-wirkungen.de/wirkungen/kaffee-und-krankheitsbilder/lebererkrankungen/.

Friedrich, Kilian, Mark Smit, Andreas Wannhoff, Christian Rupp, Sabine G. Scholl, Christoph
    Antoni, Matthias Dollinger, et al. "Coffee Consumption Protects against Progression in
    Liver Cirrhosis and Increases Long-Term Survival after Liver Transplantation." *Journal
    of Gastroenterology and Hepatology* 31, no. 8 (August 2016): 1470–75. https://doi.org
    /10.1111/jgh.13319.
Gressner, Olav A. "About Coffee, Cappuccino and Connective Tissue Growth Factor—Or
    How to Protect Your Liver!?" *Environmental Toxicology and Pharmacology* 28, no. 1 (July
    2009): 1–10. https://doi.org/10.1016/j.etap.2009.02.005.
———. "Less Smad2 Is Good for You! A Scientific Update on Coffee's Liver Benefits."
    Hepatology 50, no. 3 (September 2009): 970–78. https://doi.org/10.1002/hep.23097.
Gressner, Olav A., Birgit Lahme, Monika Siluschek, and Axel M. Gressner. "Identification
    of Paraxanthine as the Most Potent Caffeine-Derived Inhibitor of Connective Tissue
    Growth Factor Expression in Liver Parenchymal Cells." *Liver International* 29, no. 6 (July
    2009): 886–97. https://doi.org/10.1111/j.1478-3231.2009.01987.x.
Gutiérrez-Grobe, Ylse, Norberto Chávez-Tapia, Vicente Sánchez-Valle, Juan Gabriel
    Gavilanes-Espinar, Guadalupe Ponciano-Rodríguez, Misael Uribe, and Nahum Mén-
    dez-Sánchez. "High Coffee Intake Is Associated with Lower Grade Nonalcoholic Fatty
    Liver Disease: The Role of Peripheral Antioxidant Activity." *Annals of Hepatology* 11, no. 3
    (May–June 2012): 350–55. https://doi.org/10.1016/S1665-2681(19)30931-7.
Jaruvongvanich, Veeravich, Anawin Sanguankeo, Nattawat Klomjit, and Sikarin Upala.
    "Effects of Caffeine Consumption in Patients with Chronic Hepatitis C: A Systematic
    Review and Meta-analysis." *Clinics and Research in Hepatology and Gastroenterology* 41, no. 1
    (February 2017): 46–55. https://doi.org/10.1016/j.clinre.2016.05.012.
Klatsky, Arthur L., Cynthia Morton, Natalia Udaltsova, and Gary D. Friedman. "Coffee,
    Cirrhosis, and Transaminase Enzymes." *Archives of Internal Medicine* 166, no. 11 (June
    2006): 1190–95. https://doi.org/10.1001/archinte.166.11.1190.
Klemmer, Ildikó, Shintaro Yagi, and Olav A. Gressner. "Oral Application of 1,7-Dimeth-
    ylxanthine (Paraxanthine) Attenuates the Formation of Experimental Cholestatic Liver
    Fibrosis." *Hepatology Research* 41, no. 11 (November 2011): 1094–109. https://doi.org
    /10.1111/j.1872-034X.2011.00856.x.
Modi, Apurva A., Jordan J. Feld, Yoon Park, David E. Kleiner, James E. Everhart, T. Jake Liang,
    and Jay H. Hoofnagle. "Increased Caffeine Consumption Is Associated with Reduced Hepatic
    Fibrosis." *Hepatology* 51, no. 1 (January 2010): 201–9. https://doi.org/10.1002/hep.23279.
Molloy, Jeffrey W., Christopher J. Calcagno, Christopher D. Williams, Frances J. Jones, Dawn
    M. Torres, and Stephen A. Harrison. "Association of Coffee and Caffeine Consumption
    with Fatty Liver Disease, Nonalcoholic Steatohepatitis, and Degree of Hepatic Fibrosis."
    Hepatology 55, no. 2 (February 2012): 429–36. https://doi.org/10.1002/hep.24731.
Shim, Sung Gon, Dae Won Jun, Eun Kyung Kim, Waqar Khalid Saeed, Kang Nyeong
    Lee, Hang Lak Lee, Oh Young Lee, Ho Soon Choi, and Byung Chul Yoon. "Caffeine
    Attenuates Liver Fibrosis via Defective Adhesion of Hepatic Stellate Cells in Cirrhotic
    Model." *Journal of Gastroenterology and Hepatology* 28, no. 12 (December 2013): 1877–84.
    https://doi.org/10.1111/jgh.12317.
Tanida, Isei, Yoshitaka Shirasago, Ryosuke Suzuki, Ryo Abe, Takaji Wakita, Kentaro Hanada,
    and Masayoshi Fukasawa. "Inhibitory Effects of Caffeic Acid, a Coffee-Related Organic

Acid, on the Propagation of Hepatitis C Virus." *Japanese Journal of Infectious Disease* 68, no. 4 (2015): 268–75. https://doi.org/10.7883/yoken.JJID.2014.309.

Wadhawan, Manav, and Anil C. Anand. "Coffee and Liver Disease." *Journal of Clinical and Experimental Hepatology* 6, no. 1 (March 2016): 40–46. https://doi.org/10.1016/j.jceh.2016.02.003.

Xiao, Qian, Rashmi Sinha, Barry I. Graubard, and Neal D. Freedman. "Inverse Associations of Total and Decaffeinated Coffee with Liver Enzyme Levels in National Health and Nutrition Examination Survey 1999–2010." *Hepatology* 60, no. 6 (December 2014): 2091–98. https://doi.org/10.1002/hep.27367.

3.2 Healthy Nutrition and Health-Promoting Dietary Supplements Using the Example of the Twelve Vital Fields

Béliveau, Richard, and Denis Gingras. *Krebszellen mögen keine Himbeeren. Nahrungsmittel gegen Krebs. Das Immunsystem stärken und gezielt vorbeugen* [Foods to fight cancer: What to eat to reduce your risk]. Munich: Goldmann Verlag, 2019.

Budwig, Johanna. *Krebs, das Problem und die Lösung. Die Dokumentation* [Cancer, the problem and the solution: The documentation]. N.p.: Sensei Verlag, 2010.

———. *Die Original-Öl-Eiweiß-Kost. Das Grundlagenbuch* [The original oil protein diet: The basics]. The Foundation's edition. Munich: Knaur Verlag, 2017.

CSIRO. "Refrigerated Storage of Perishable Foods." Updated September 9, 2021. https://www.csiro.au/en/research/production/food/Refrigerating-foods.

Dei Cas, Michele, and Riccardo Ghidoni. "Dietary Curcumin: Correlation between Bioavailability and Health Potential." In "Dietary Curcumin and Human Health," ed. Riccardo Ghidoni, Mariarosa Anna Beatrice Melone, and Chiara Terracciano, special issue, *Nutrients* 11, no. 9 (September 2019): 2147. https://doi.org/10.3390/nu11092147.

Dittrich-Opitz, Christian. *Mitochondrien. Mehr Lebensenergie durch gesunde Zellkraftwerke* [Mitochondria: More vital energy thanks to healthy cell power plants]. Rossdorf: Hans-Nietsch-Verlag, 2017.

Drevs, Joachim. *Integrative Onkologie. Definition, Inhalte, Bedeutung* [Integrative oncology: Definition, contents, significance]. Berlin: De Gruyter Verlag, 2020.

Know, Lee. *Die Mito-Medizin. Wie Sie Ihre Zellkraftwerke schützen, Krankheiten heilen und lange leben. Gesunde Mitochondrien, gesunder Körper* [Mitochondria and the future of medicine]. Kirchzarten: VAK Verlag, 2018.

Longo, Valter. *Iss dich jung. Wissenschaftlich erprobte Ernährung für ein gesundes und langes Leben. Die Longevità-Diät* [Eat yourself young: Scientifically proven nutrition for a healthy and long life—the longevity diet]. Munich: Goldmann Verlag, 2018.

———. *The Longevity Diet: Discover the New Science Behind Stem Cell Activation and Regeneration to Slow Aging, Fight Disease, and Optimize Weight*. New York: Avery, 2018. Pennsylvania State University. "News." news.psu.edu.

Schlenga, Suzanne. "Fast jeder Patient schluckt zu viele Pillen" [Almost every patient swallows too many pills]. *Westfalenpost*, December 28, 2013. https://www.wp.de/staedte/herdecke-wetter/fast-jeder-patient-schluckt-zu-viele-pillen-id8813346.html.

Schreiber, David Servan. *Das Anti-Krebs Buch. Was uns schützt: Vorbeugen und Nachsorgen mit natürlichen Mitteln* [The anticancer book: What protects us—prevention and aftercare with natural means]. Munich: Goldmann Verlag, 2010.

Sheffield Chamber of Commerce and Industry. "Freeze-Dried Fruit Does Retain Its Goodness." September 10, 2013. https://www.scci.org.uk/news/freeze-dried-fruit-does
-retain-its-goodness/.

Wark, Chris. *Chris Beat Cancer: A Comprehensive Plan for Healing Naturally.* New York: Hay
House, 2018.

Zentrum der Gesundheit [The health center]. www.zentrum-der-gesundheit.de.

Zentrum der Gesundheit [The health center]. "Kohlgemüse: Die Sorten und die gesund-
heitlichen Aspekte" [Cabbage vegetables: The varieties and the health aspects]. https://
www.zentrum-der-gesundheit.de/heilkraft-von-kohl.html.

3.3 Water: An Elixir of Life

Batmanghelidj, F. *Sie sind nicht krank, Sie sind durstig! Heilung von innen mit Wasser und Salz*
[Water: For health, for healing, for life—you're not sick, you're thirsty!]. Kirchzarten:
VAK Verlag, 2003.

Class, Alexander. "Strömungsberechnungen für VortexPower AG" [Flow calculations for
VortexPower]. Unpublished report prepared for VitaVortex AG, 2013. (Unpublished
measurement protocols, experimentally measured and made on assignment for the
company VitaVortex AG, received directly from the author.)

Pollack, Gerald H. *Cells, Gels and the Engines of Life: A New, Unifying Approach to Cell Function.*
Seattle: Ebner and Sons, 2001.

———. *Wasser. Viel mehr als H2O* [Water: Much more than H_2O]. Kirchzarten: VAK Verlag, 2014.

Sheldrake, Rupert. *Das schöpferische Universum. Die Theorie des Morphogenetischen Feldes* [The creative universe: The theory of the morphogenetic field]. Berlin: Ullstein Buchverlage, 1993.

3.4 Oxygen, Breathing, and Cancer Growth

Francia, Luisa. *Beschützt, bewahrt, geborgen. Wie magischer Schutz wirklich funktioniert* [Protected,
preserved, safe: How magical protection really works]. Berlin: Ullstein Verlag, 2010.

Kreutzer, Franz. *Intravenöse Sauerstofftherapie (IOT). Oxyvenierungstherapie nach Dr. Regelsberger
in Theorie und Praxis. Von den Anfängen bis in die Gegenwart* [Intravenous oxygen therapy
(IOT): Oxyvenation therapy according to Dr. Regelsberger in theory and practice—from
the beginnings to the present day]. N.p.: Deutsche Gesellschaft für Oxyvenierungstherapie e.V. [German society for oxyvenation therapy], 2013.

Petrova, Varvara, Margherita Annicchiarico-Petruzzelli, Gerry Melino, and Ivano Amelio.
"The Hypoxic Tumour Environment." *Oncogenesis* 7 (2018): 10. https://doi.org/10.1038
/s41389-017-0011-9.

Regelsberger, Helmut Siegfried. *Oxyvenierungstherapie in Wissenschaft und Praxis* [Oxyvena-
tion therapy in science and practice]. Stuttgart: Haug Verlag, 1976.

Segatz, Helga. "Zwerchfellatmung" [Diaphragmatic breathing]. Atmen mit Helga Segatz
[Breathing with Helga Segatz], March 27, 2009. https://www.atemmassage.de
/atemerfahrung/allgemeines-zum-atem/zwerchfellatmung.

Von Ardenne, Manfred. *Wo hilft Sauerstoff-Mehrschritt-Therapie? Erster schneller Weg zur
anhaltenden Steigerung der Energie im menschlichen Organismus* [Where does oxygen multistep therapy help? The first quick way for sustainably increasing energy in the human
organism]. Munich: Urban und Fischer Verlag, 1989.

3.5. Maintaining Intestinal Health

Banerjee, Sagarika, Tian Tian, Zhi Wei, Natalie Shih, Michael D. Feldman, James C. Alwine, George Coukos, and Erle S. Robertson. "The Ovarian Cancer Oncobiome." *Oncotarget* 8, no. 22 (March 2017): 36225–45. https://www.doi.org/10.18632/oncotarget.16717.

Hung, Ivan F. N., and Benjamin C. Y. Wong. "Assessing the Risks and Benefits of Treating *Helicobacter pylori* Infection." *Therapeutic Advances in Gasteroenterology* 2, no. 3 (May 2009): 141–47. https://doi.org/10.1177/1756283X08100279.

Iida, Noriho, Amiran Dzutsev, C. Andrew Stewart, Loretta Smith, Nicolas Bouladoux, Rebecca A. Weingarten, Daniel A. Molina, et al. "Commensal Bacteria Control Cancer Response to Therapy by Modulating the Tumor Microenvironment." *Science* 342, no. 6161 (November 2013): 967–70. https://doi.org/10.1126/science.1240527.

Marschalek, Julian, Alex Farr, Marie-Louise Marschalek, Konrad J. Domig, Wolfgang Kneifel, Christian F. Singer, Herbert Kiss, and Ljubomir Petricevic. "Influence of Orally Administered Probiotic *Lactobacillus* Strains on Vaginal Microbiota in Women with Breast Cancer during Chemotherapy: A Randomized Placebo-Controlled Double-Blinded Pilot Study." *Breast Care* 12, no. 5 (October 2017): 335–39. https://doi.org/10.1159/000478994.

Martin, Alyce M., Julian M. Yabut, Jocelyn M. Choo, Amanda J. Page, Emily W. Sun, Claire F. Jessup, Steve L. Wesselingh, et al. "The Gut Microbiome Regulates Host Glucose Homeostasis via Peripheral Serotonin." *Proceedings of the National Academy of Sciences* 116, no. 40 (October 2019): 19802–804. https://doi.org/10.1073/pnas.1909311116.

MyMicrobiome. Accessed 2021. www.mymicrobiome.info.

Valles-Colomer, Mireia, Gwen Falony, Youssef Darzi, Ettje F. Tigchelaar, Jun Wang, Raul Y. Tito, Carmen Schiweck, et al. "The Neuroactive Potential of the Human Gut Microbiota in Quality of Life and Depression." *Nature Microbiology* 4 (April 2019): 623–32. https://doi.org/10.1038/s41564-018-0337-x.

Vancamelbeke, Maaike, and Séverine Vermeire. "The Intestinal Barrier: A Fundamental Role in Health and Disease." *Expert Review of Gastroenterology and Hepatology* 11, no. 9 (2017): 821–34. https://doi.org/10.1080/17474124.2017.1343143.

3.6 Stress

Banerjee, S., R. Califano, J. Corral, E. de Azambuja, L. De Mattos-Arruda, V. Guarneri, M. Hutka, et al. "Professional Burnout in European Young Oncologists: Results of the European Society for Medical Oncology (ESMO) Young Oncologists Committee Burnout Survey." *Annals of Oncology* 28, no. 7 (July 2017): 1590–96. https://doi.org/10.1093/annonc/mdx196.

Fuchs, Reinhard, and Markus Gerber, eds. *Handbuch Stressregulation und Sport* [Handbook on stress regulation and sport]. Springer Reference Psychologie. Heidelberg/Berlin: Springer Verlag, 2018.

Hapke, U., U. E. Masks, C. Scheidt-Nave, L. Bode, R. Schlack, and M. A. Busch. "Chronischer Stress bei Erwachsenen in Deutschland. Ergebnisse der Studie zur Gesundheit Erwachsener in Deutschland (DEGS1)" [Chronic stress among adults in Germany: Results of the German Health Interview and Examination Survey for Adults (DEGS1)]. *Bundesgesundheitsblatt - Gesundheitsforschung - Gesundheitsschutz* 56 (May 2013): 749–54. https://doi.org/10.1007/s00103-013-1690-9.

Küchler, Thomas, Beate Bestmann, Stefanie Rappat, Doris Henne-Bruns, and Sharon Wood-Dauphinee. "Impact of Psychotherapeutic Support for Patients with Gastrointestinal Cancer Undergoing Surgery: 10-Year Survival Results of a Randomized Trial." *Journal of Clinical Oncology* 25, no. 19 (July 2007): 2702–8. https://doi.org/10.1200/JCO.2006.08.2883.

Medisauskaite, Asta, and Caroline Kamau. "Prevalence of Oncologists in Distress: Systematic Review and Meta-analysis." *Psycho-Oncology* 26, no. 11 (November 2017): 1732–40. https://doi.org/10.1002/pon.4382.

Morgan, Graeme, Robyn Ward, and Michael Barton. "The Contribution of Cytotoxic Chemotherapy to 5-Year Survival in Adult Malignancies." *Clinical Oncology* 16, no. 8 (December 2004): 549–60. https://doi.org/10.1016/j.clon.2004.06.007.

Reps, Paul. *Ohne Worte – ohne Schweigen. 101 Zen-Geschichten* [Without words—without silence: 101 Zen stories]. Munich: O.W. Barth Verlag, 1989.

Rosa, Hartmut. *Beschleunigung. Die Veränderung der Zeitstrukturen in der Moderne* [Acceleration: Changing time structures in the modern age]. Frankfurt: Suhrkamp Verlag, 2005.

Schmid, Gary Bruno. *Selbstheilung durch Vorstellungskraft* [Self-healing by imagination]. Heidelberg/Berlin: Springer Verlag, 2011.

Simonton, Oscar Carl. *Auf dem Wege der Besserung. Schritte zur körperlichen und spirituellen Heilung* [On the road to recovery: Steps to physical and spiritual healing]. Reinbek: Rowohlt Verlag, 2013.

Simonton, Oscar Carl, Stephanie Matthews Simonton, and James Creighton. *Wieder gesund werden. Eine Anleitung zur Aktivierung der Selbstheilungskräfte für Krebspatienten und ihre Angehörigen. Übungen zur Entspannung und Visualisierung nach der Simonton-Methode* [Getting well again: A step-by-step, self-help guide to overcoming cancer for patients and their families]. Reinbek: Rowohlt Verlag, 2001.

Tolle, Eckhart. *Jetzt! Die Kraft der Gegenwart. Ein Leitfaden zum spirituellen Erwachen* [The power of now: A guide to spiritual enlightenment]. Bielefeld: Kamphausen Verlag, 2010.

Turner, Kelly. *9 Wege in ein krebsfreies Leben. Wahre Geschichten von geheilten Menschen* [Radical remission: Surviving cancer against all odds—the nine key factors that can make a real difference]. Munich: Irisiana Verlag, 2015.

Währborg, Peter. *Stress och den nya ohälsan* [Stress and the new unhealthiness]. Stockholm: Natur och Kultur, 2002.

Yawger, N. S. "Emotions as the Cause of Rapid and Sudden Death." *Archives of Neurology and Psychiatry* (1936): 875–79.

3.7 Sugar: Cancer Driver of the First Order

Donner, Susanne. "Warum viele in die Süßstofffalle tappen" [Why so many fall into the trap of sweeteners]. *Die Welt*, April 28, 2014. https://www.welt.de/gesundheit/article127380003/Warum-viele-in-die-Suessstofffalle-tappen.html.

Soffritti, Morando, Michela Padovani, Eva Tibaldi, Laura Falcioni, Fabiana Manservisi, and Fiorella Belpoggi. "The Carcinogenic Effects of Aspartame: The Urgent Need for Regulatory Re-evaluation." *American Journal of Industrialized Medicine* 57, no. 4 (April 2014): 383–97. https://doi.org/10.1002/ajim.22296.

Suez, Jotham, Tal Korem, David Zeevi, Gili Zilberman-Schapira, Christoph A. Thaiss, Ori
    Maza, David Israeli, et al. "Artificial Sweeteners Induce Glucose Intolerance by Altering
    the Gut Microbiota." *Nature* 514 (September 2014): 181–86. https://doi.org/10.1038
    /nature13793.
Winters, Nasha, and Jess Higgins Kelley. *Stoffwechsel in Balance. Krebs ohne Chance* [The met-
    abolic approach to cancer: Integrating deep nutrition, the ketogenic diet, and nontoxic
    bio-individualized therapies]. Munich: Riva Verlag, 2018.

3.8 The Shift of the Immune System
Janssen, Louise M. E., Emma F. Ramsay, Craig D. Logsdon, and Willem W. Overwijk. "The
    Immune System in Cancer Metastasis: Friend or Foe?" *Journal for ImmunoTherapy of
    Cancer* 5, no. 1 (Oct 2017): 79. https://doi.org/10.1186/s40425-017-0283-9.
Ji, Jianguang, Kristina Sundquist, Yi Ning, Kenneth S. Kendler, Jan Sundquist, and Xiangning
    Chen. "Incidence of Cancer in Patients with Schizophrenia and Their First-Degree
    Relatives: A Population-Based Study in Sweden." *Schizophrenia Bulletin* 39, no. 3 (May
    2013): 527–36. https://doi.org/10.1093/schbul/sbs065.

3.9 Mitochondria: Power Plants of the Cells
Béliveau, Richard, and Denis Gingras. *Krebszellen mögen keine Himbeeren. Nahrungsmittel gegen
    Krebs. Das Immunsystem stärken und gezielt vorbeugen* [Foods to fight cancer: What to eat to
    reduce your risk]. Munich: Goldmann Verlag, 2019.
Buck, Katharina, Aida Karina Zaineddin, Susen Becker, Anika Hüsing, Rudolf Kaaks, Jakob
    Linseisen, Dieter Flesch-Janys, and Jenny Chang-Claude. "Serum Enterolactone and
    Prognosis of Postmenopausal Breast Cancer." *Journal of Clinical Oncology* 29, no. 28
    (October 2011): 3730–38. https://doi.org/10.1200/JCO.2011.34.6478.
Dittrich-Opitz, Christian. *Mitochondrien. Mehr Lebensenergie durch gesunde Zellkraftwerke*
    [Mitochondria: More vital energy thanks to healthy cell power plants]. Rossdorf:
    Hans-Nietsch-Verlag, 2017.
Drevs, Joachim. *Integrative Onkologie. Definition, Inhalte, Bedeutung* [Integrative oncology:
    Definition, contents, significance]. Berlin: De Gruyter Verlag, 2020.
Know, Lee. *Die Mito-Medizin. Wie Sie Ihre Zellkraftwerke schützen, Krankheiten heilen und lange
    leben. Gesunde Mitochondrien, gesunder Körper* [Mitochondria and the future of medicine].
    Kirchzarten: VAK Verlag, 2018.
Ray, Anasuya, Smreti Vasudevan, and Suparna Sengupta. "6-Shogaol Inhibits Breast Cancer
    Cells and Stem Cell–Like Spheroids by Modulation of Notch Signaling Pathway and
    Induction of Autophagic Cell Death." *PLOS ONE* 10, no. 9 (September 2015): e0137614.
    https://doi.org/10.1371/journal.pone.0137614.
Seyfried, Thomas N. *Cancer as a Metabolic Disease: On the Origin, Management, and Prevention
    of Cancer*. New York: Wiley, 2012.

3.10 The Acid-Base Balance
Pischinger, Alfred. *Das System der Grundregulation. Grundlagen einer ganzheitsbiologischen
    Medizin* [The system of basic regulation: Fundamentals of holistic biological medicine].
    Stuttgart: F. W. Haug Verlag, 2010.

Van Limburg-Stirum, John. *Moderne Säure-Basen-Medizin. Physiologie – Diagnostik – Therapie* [Modern acid-base medicine: Physiology—diagnostics—therapy]. Berlin: Hippokrates GmbH, 2008.

Yeo, Marie, Dong-Kyu Kim, Young-Bae Kim, Tae Young Oh, Jong-Eun Lee, Sung Won Cho, Hugh Chul Kim, and Ki-Baik Hahm. "Selective Induction of Apoptosis with Proton Pump Inhibitors in Gastric Cancer." *Clinical Cancer Research* 10, no. 24 (December 2004): 8687–96. https://doi.org/10.1158/1078-0432.CCR-04-1065.

3.11 Healing and Preventing Infections

Fachgesellschaft für Ernährungstherapie und Prävention [Society for nutritional therapy and prevention]. "Chronische Entzündungen (Inflammation) – Symptombild und Ernährungstherapie" [Chronic inflammation—symptoms and nutritional therapy]. Last updated May 10, 2022. https://fet-ev.eu/entzuendungen-symptombild.

Jensen, Gitte. "Cerule Scientific Advisory Board: Gitte Jensen, PhD." My Stem Cell Power. https://mystemcellpower.com/business/gitte-jensen-phd.html.

———, ed. *Pleomorphic Microbes in Health and Disease: Proceedings of the First Annual Symposium Held June 18–19, 1999 in Montreal, Quebec, Canada*. Port Dover, Ontario: Holger N.I.S., 1999.

3.12 Chronic Inflammation: Silent Inflammation

Balkwill, Frances, Kellie A. Charles, and Alberto Mantovani. "Smoldering and Polarized Inflammation in the Initiation and Promotion of Malignant Disease." *Cancer Cell* 7, no. 3 (March 2005): 211–17. https://doi.org/10.1016/j.ccr.2005.02.013.

Singh, Nitin, Deepak Baby, Jagadish Prasad Rajguru, Pankaj B. Patil, Savita S. Thakkannavar, and Veena Bhojaraj Pujari. "Inflammation and Cancer." *Annals of African Medicine* 18, no. 3 (July–September 2019): 121–26. https://doi.org/10.4103/aam.aam_56_18.

Stix, Gary. "A Malignant Flame: Understanding Chronic Inflammation, Which Contributes to Heart Disease, Alzheimer's and a Variety of Other Ailments, May Be a Key to Unlocking the Mysteries of Cancer." *Scientific American* 297, no. 1 (July 2007): 60–67. https://doi.org/10.1038/scientificamerican0707-60.

Chapter 4. Balance: Everything in Flux

Turner, Kelly. *9 Wege in ein krebsfreies Leben. Wahre Geschichten von geheilten Menschen* [Radical remission: Surviving cancer against all odds—the nine key factors that can make a real difference]. Munich: Irisiana Verlag, 2015.

Chapter 5. Strategies of Biologically Based Complementary Oncology

Barkleit, Gerhard. "Scheitern eines innovativen Ansatzes. Manfred von Ardenne und die Krebs-Mehrschritt-Therapie" [Failure of an innovative approach: Manfred von Ardenne and cancer multi-step therapy]. *Deutsches Ärzteblatt International* 102, no. 6 (February 2005): 344–48. https://www.aerzteblatt.de/int/article.asp?id=45331.

Coley Nauts, Helen, and John R. McLaren. "Coley Toxins: The First Century." In *Consensus on Hyperthermia for the 1990s: Clinical Practice in Cancer Treatment*, edited by Haim I. Bicher, John R. McLaren, and Giuseppe M. Pigliucci, 483–500. New York: Springer, 1990.

Datta, Niloy R., H. Petra Kok, Hans Crezee, Udo S. Gaipl, and Stephan Bodis. "Integrating Loco-Regional Hyperthermia into the Current Oncology Practice: SWOT and TOWS Analyses." *Frontiers in Oncology* 10 (June 2020): 819. https://doi.org/10.3389/fonc.2020.00819.

Flashar, Hellmut. *Hippokrates. Meister der Heilkunst* [Hippocrates: Master of medicine]. Munich: CH Beck Verlag, 2016.

Hauser, Ross A., and Marion A. Hauser. *Treating Cancer with Insulin Potentiation Therapy.* Self-published, Beulah Land Press, 2002.

Meyers, Bryant A. *PEMF: The 5th Element of Health.* Self-published, Balboa Press, 2013.

Moore, Wendy. "The Edwin Smith Papyrus." *BMJ* 342 (March 2011): d1598. https://doi.org/10.1136/bmj.d1598.

Szasz, Andras, Nora Szasz, and Oliver Szasz. *Oncothermia: Principles and Practices.* Berlin: Springer Verlag, 2011.

Thomas, Melanie B., and Andrew X. Zhu. "Hepatocellular Carcinoma: The Need for Progress." *Journal of Clinical Oncology* 23, no. 13 (May 2005): 2892–99. https://doi.org/10.1200/JCO.2005.03.196.

Vadalà, Maria, Julio Cesar Morales-Medina, Annamaria Vallelunga, Beniamino Palmieri, Carmen Laurino, and Tommaso Iannitti. "Mechanisms and Therapeutic Effectiveness of Pulsed Electromagnetic Field Therapy in Oncology." *Cancer Medicine* 5, no. 11 (November 2016): 3128–39. https://doi.org/10.1002/cam4.861.

Chapter 6. Cancer Therapies: Outside the Box

Derry, David M. *Breast Cancer and Iodine.* Self-published, Trafford Publishing, 2001.

Giovannucci, Edward, Yan Liu, Eric B. Rimm, Bruce W. Hollis, Charles S. Fuchs, Meir J. Stampfer, and Walter C. Willett. "Prospective Study of Predictors of Vitamin D Status and Cancer Incidence and Mortality in Men." *Journal of the National Cancer Institute* 98, no. 7 (April 2006): 451–59. https://doi.org/10.1093/jnci/djj101.

Gorham, Edward D., Cedric F. Garland, Frank C. Garland, William B. Grant, Sharif B. Mohr, Martin Lipkin, Harold L. Newmark, Edward Giovannucci, Melissa Wei, and Michael F. Holick. "Vitamin D and Prevention of Colorectal Cancer." *Journal of Steroid Biochemistry and Molecular Biology* 97, nos. 1–2 (October 2005): 179–94. https://doi.org/10.1016/j.jsbmb.2005.06.018.

Grant, William B. "An Estimate of Premature Cancer Mortality in the U.S. Due to Inadequate Doses of Solar Ultraviolet-B Radiation." *Cancer* 94, no. 6 (March 2002): 1867–75. https://doi.org/10.1002/cncr.10427.

Gröber, Uwe. *Arzneimittel und Mikronährstoffe. Medikationsorientierte Supplementierung* [Drugs and micronutrients: Medication-oriented supplementation]. 4th ed. Stuttgart: Wissenschaftliche Verlagsgesellschaft, 2018.

———. *Orthomolekulare Medizin* [Orthomolecular medicine]. Stuttgart: Wissenschaftliche Verlagsgesellschaft, 2008.

Kelley, Robin K., and Andrew H. Ko. "Erlotinib in the Treatment of Advanced Pancreatic Cancer." *Biologics: Targets and Therapy* 2, no. 1 (2008): 83–95. https://doi.org/10.2147/BTT.S1832.

Kienle, Gunver. "Misteltherapie bei Krebs. Was ist belegt, was nicht?" [Mistletoe therapy for cancer: What is proven, what is not?]. *Gynäkologie und Geburtshilfe* 11 (2009): 52–53. https://www.ifaemm.de/Abstract/PDFs/GK09_3.pdf.

Lamprecht, Manfred, Simon Bogner, Kurt Steinbauer, Burkhard Schuetz, Joachim F. Greil-
berger, Bettina Leber, Bernhard Wagner, et al. "Effects of Zeolite Supplementation on
Parameters of Intestinal Barrier Integrity, Inflammation, Redoxbiology and Performance
in Aerobically Trained Subjects." *Journal of the International Society of Sports Nutrition* 12
(October 2015): 40. https://doi.org/10.1186/s12970-015-0101-z.

Longo, Valter. *Iss dich jung. Wissenschaftlich erprobte Ernährung für ein gesundes und langes Leben.
Die Longevità-Diät* [Eat yourself young: Scientifically proven nutrition for a healthy and
long life—the longevity diet]. Munich: Goldmann Verlag, 2018.

Mastinu, Andrea, Amit Kumar, Giuseppina Maccarinelli, Sara Anna Bonini, Marika Premoli,
Francesca Aria, Alessandra Gianoncelli, and Maurizio Memo. "Zeolite Clinoptilolite:
Therapeutic Virtues of an Ancient Mineral." *Molecules* 24, no. 8 (April 2019): 1517.
https://doi.org/10.3390/molecules24081517.

Paepke, Daniela. "Komplementärmedizin für eine bessere Lebensqualität" [Complementary
medicine for a better quality of life]. *Im Fokus Onkologie* 23, no. 4 (2020): 66–70. https://
doi.org/10.1007/s15015-020-2424-0.

———. "Die Misteltherapie in der Onkologie" [Mistletoe therapy in oncology]. *Im Fokus
Onkologie* 21, no. 3 (2018): 64–68. https://doi.org/10.1007/s15015-018-3855-8.

Schön, Christiane, and Frank Bayer. "Enzympräparate unter der Lupe" [Enzyme preparations
under the magnifying glass]. *Deutsche Apotheker Zeitung* 22 (May 2013): 71. https://www
.deutsche-apotheker-zeitung.de/daz-az/2013/daz-22-2013/enzympraeparate-unter-der-lupe.

Simonton, Oscar Carl. *Auf dem Wege der Besserung. Schritte zur körperlichen und spirituellen
Heilung* [On the road to recovery: Steps to physical and spiritual healing]. Reinbek:
Rowohlt Verlag, 2013.

Tipping, Colin. *Ich vergebe. Der radikale Abschied vom Opferdasein* [Radical forgiveness: Making
room for the miracle]. Bielefeld: Kamphausen Verlag, 2010.

Torremante, P. "Mastopathie, Mammakarzinom und Jodlactone" [Mastopathy, breast cancer
and iodolactone]. *Deutsche Medizinische Wochenschrift* 129, no. 12 (2004): 641–46. https://
doi.org/10.1055/s-2004-820575.

Tröger, Wilfried, D. Galun, Marcus Reif, Agnes Schumann, Nikola Stanković, and Miroslav
Milicevic. "Lebensqualität von Patienten mit fortgeschrittenem Pankreaskarzinom
unter Misteltherapie in einer randomisierten Überlebenszeitstudie" [Quality of life of
patients with advanced pancreatic cancer during treatment with mistletoe: A randomized
controlled trial]. *Deutsches Ärzteblatt International* 111, nos. 29–30 (July 2014): 493–502.
https://doi.org/10.3238/arztebl.2014.0493.

Turner, Kelly, and Tracy White. *Radical Hope: 10 Key Healing Factors from Exceptional Survivors
of Cancer and Other Diseases*. New York: Hay House, 2020.

Vitalpilze. Naturheilkraft mit Tradition neu entdeckt [Medicinal mushrooms: Traditional natural
healing rediscovered]. N.p.: printed by Gesellschaft für Vitalpilze e.V. [Community for
medicinal mushrooms science], 2014.

Weißenborn, Anke, Nadiya Bakhiya, Irmela Demuth, Anke Ehlers, Monika Ewald, Birgit
Niemann, Klaus Richter, et al. "Höchstmengen für Vitamine und Mineralstoffe in
Nahrungsergänzungsmitteln" [Maximum levels for vitamins and minerals in food
supplements]. *Journal für Verbraucherschutz und Lebensmittelsicherheit* 13 (January 2018):
25–39. https://doi.org/10.1007/s00003-017-1140-y.

Kabat-Zinn, Jon. *Gesund durch Meditation* [Healthy through Meditation]. 6th ed. Munich: O. W. Barth Verlag, 2011.

Treatment with Medicines Without Approval

Corsello, Steven M., Rohith T. Nagari, Ryan D. Spangler, Jordan Rossen, Mustafa Kocak, Jordan G. Bryan, Ranad Humeidi, et al. "Discovering the Anticancer Potential of Non-oncology Drugs by Systematic Viability Profiling." *Nature Cancer* 1 (2020): 235–48. https://doi.org/10.1038/s43018-019-0018-6.

Dowideit, Anette. "Leben hat seinen preis" [Life has its price]. *Die Welt am Sonntag*, November 13, 2016. https://www.mamazone.de/fileadmin/downloads/Aktuelles/2016/artikel_welt_am_sonntag_friesen.pdf.

Ekinci, Elmira, Sagar Rohondia, Raheel Khan, and Qingping P. Dou. "Repurposing Disulfiram as an Anti-Cancer Agent: Updated Review on Literature and Patents." *Recent Patents on Anti-Cancer Drug Discovery* 14, no. 2 (2019): 113–32. https://doi.org/10.2174/1574892814666190514104035.

Friesen, Claudia, Inis Hormann, Mareike Roscher, Iduna Fichtner, Andreas Alt, Ralf Hilger, Klaus-Michael Debatin, and Erich Miltner. "Opioid Receptor Activation Triggering Downregulation of cAMP Improves Effectiveness of Anti-Cancer Drugs in Treatment of Glioblastoma." *Cell Cycle* 13, no. 10 (March 2014): 1560–70. https://doi.org/10.4161/cc.28493.

Friesen, Claudia, Mareike Roscher, Andreas Alt, and Erich Miltner. "Methadone: Commonly Used as Maintenance Medication for Outpatient Treatment of Opioid Dependence, Kills Leukemia Cells and Overcomes Chemoresistance." *Cancer Research* 68, no. 15 (August 2008): 6059–64. https://doi.org/10.1158/0008-5472.CAN-08-1227.

Friesen, Claudia, Mareike Roscher, Inis Hormann, Iduna Fichtner, Andreas Alt, Ralf A. Hilger, Klaus-Michael Debatin, and Erich Miltner. "Cell Death Sensitization of Leukemia Cells by Opioid Receptor Activation." *Oncotarget* 4 (2013): 655–90. https://doi.org/10.18632/oncotarget.952.

Huang, Wuqing, Jan Sundquist, Kristina Sundquist, Jianguang Ji. "Phosphodiesterase-5 Inhibitors Use and Risk for Mortality and Metastases among Male Patients with Colorectal Cancer." *Nature Communications* 11 (2020): 3191. https://doi.org/10.1038/s41467-020-17028-4.

McLelland, Jane. *Den Krebs aushungern, ohne selbst zu hungern. Die außergewöhnliche Überlebensgeschichte einer mutigen Frau und eine Entdeckung, die das Leben von Millionen Menschen verändern könnte* [Starve cancer, without starving yourself: One courageous woman's extraordinary survival story and a discovery that could change the lives of millions]. Kirchzarten: VAK Verlag, 2020.

Moorjani, Anita. *Heilung im Licht. Wie ich durch eine Nahtoderfahrung den Krebs besiegte und neu geboren wurde* [Healing in light: How I beat cancer and was reborn through a near-death experience]. Munich: Goldmann Verlag, 2015.

Novalis [Georg Philipp Friedrich von Hardenberg]. "Hymne an die nacht 5" [Hymns to the night 5]. In *Novalis Werke* [Works of Novalis]. Munich: C. H. Beck Verlag, 1969.

Tang, Jing, Zhijie Li, Lan Lu, and Chi Hin Cho. "β-Adrenergic System, a Backstage Manipulator Regulating Tumour Progression and Drug Target in Cancer Therapy." *Seminars in Cancer Biology* 23, no. 6, part B (December 2013): 533–42. https://doi.org/10.1016/j.semcancer.2013.08.009.

Tołoczko-Iwaniuk, Natalia, Dorota Dziemiańczyk-Pakieła, Beata Klaudia Nowaszewska, Katarzyna Celińska-Janowicz, and Wojciech Miltyk. "Celecoxib in Cancer Therapy and Prevention—Review." *Current Drug Targets* 20, no. 3 (March 2019): 302–15. https://doi .org/10.2174/1389450119666180803121737.

Zi, Fuming, Huapu Zi, Yi Li, Jingsong He, Qingzhi Shi, and Zhen Cai. "Metformin and Cancer: An Existing Drug for Cancer Prevention and Therapy." *Oncology Letters* 15, no. 1 (January 2018): 683–90. https://doi.org/10.3892/ol.2017.7412.

ILT and Meditations

Chödrön, Pema. *Die Weisheit der Ausweglosigkeit* [Comfortable with uncertainty: 108 teachings on cultivating fearlessness and compassion]. Freiburg: Arbor Verlag, 2012.

Hay, Louise. *Gesundheit für Körper und Seele* [You can heal your life]. Berlin: Ullstein Verlag Berlin, 2010.

Martinez, Mario. *The MindBody Code: How to Change the Beliefs that Limit your Health, Longevity, and Success*. Louisville, CO: Sounds True, 2016.

Nath Hanh, Thich. *Das Wunder der Achtsamkeit* [The miracle of mindfulness]. Bielefeld: Theseus Verlag, 2009.

Tipping, Colin. *Radical Forgiveness: A Revolutionary Five-Stage Process to Heal Relationships, Let Go of Anger and Blame, and Find Peace in Any Situation*. Louisville, CO: Sounds True, 2010.

Tolle, Eckhart. *Jetzt! Die Kraft der Gegenwart. Ein Leitfaden zum spirituellen Erwachen* [The power of now: A guide to spiritual enlightenment]. Bielefeld: Kamphausen Verlag, 2010.

Turner, Kelly. *9 Wege in ein krebsfreies Leben. Wahre Geschichten von geheilten Menschen* [Radical remission: Surviving cancer against all odds—the nine key factors that can make a real difference]. Munich: Irisiana Verlag, 2015.

Turner, Kelly, and Tracy White. *Hoffnung auf ein krebsfreies Leben. Die 10 Schlüsselfaktoren der Heilung* [Radical hope: 10 key healing factors from exceptional survivors of cancer and other diseases]. Munich: Irisiana Verlag, 2021.

Winters, Nasha, and Jess Higgins Kelley. "Kapitel 12. Seelisches und emotionales Wohlbe-finden: die stärkste Medizin" [Chapter 12: Mental and emotional wellbeing—cultivating the most powerful medicine of all]. In *Stoffwechsel in Balance. Krebs ohne Chance* [The metabolic approach to cancer: Integrating deep nutrition, the ketogenic diet, and nontoxic bio-individualized therapies]. Munich: Riva Verlag, 2018.

Index

Note: Page numbers in italics refer to figures. Page numbers followed by *t* refer to tables. Page numbers preceded by ci refer to the color insert section.

5-aminolevulinic acid (5ALA), 211
6-shogaol, 46

abdominal breathing, 86, 143
    See also breathing
acacia fibers
    for blood glucose regulation, 197
    for gut health, 46, 59, 191
accepting what is, in mindfulness training, 192, 227
acerola cherries, vitamin C in, 66
acesulfame-K (sugar substitute), 113
acetylsalicylic acid
    anti inflammatory qualities, 152
    blood-thinning qualities, 220
acid–base balance, 135–145
    biochemistry of, 136–39
    complementary deacidification therapies,
        142–45, 202–3
    dietary recommendations, 73–76, 74t, 75t
    immune system shifts and, 116
    importance for inflammation and cancer, 140
    live blood analysis, 139, 176, ci2
    as one of the twelve vital fields, 9
    organ hypoxia effects on, 83
    overacidification and measurement methods,
        141–42
    overview, 135–36
acid–base reactions, 136–37, 138
acid-forming foods, 74, 75
acidification. *See* hyperacidity
acids
    biochemistry of, 136–39
    as toxins, 32
acute infections, 147
    See also infections
acute inflammation
    blood tests for measuring, 153

    as protective measure of infections, 145–49
    transforming chronic inflammation into, 151–52
acute vs. chronic acidosis, 135–36
acute vs. chronic stress, 99
    See also stress
adaptability, importance of, 224–25
adaptogens, 199–201
adhesion molecules, 89
adsorption detoxification therapies, 184–85
affirmations, 123–25, 228–29, ci7
    See also healing meditations
aging
    alpha lipoic acid benefits, 132
    lack of oxygen related to, 83
    mitochondrial damage linked to, 130–31
    strategies for activating mitochondria, 131–34
ajoene, 41
Akhenaten (pharaoh), 28
ALA (alpha-linolenic acid), 55, 56
alcohol, breakdown in the liver, 32
alkaline baths, 145
alkaline powders, 76, 203
alkaline procaine infusions, 182–83, 203
allicin
    Nf-Kappa-B inhibition by, 152
    in the onion family, 40–41
allostasis, 97
aloe vera, for gut health, 191
alpha-linolenic acid (ALA), 55, 56
alpha lipoic acid
    acid–base balance benefits, 203
    detoxifying effect of, 183
    mitochondria-strengthening benefits of, 72, 132
alternative cancer therapies. *See* complementary
    oncology; outside-the-box cancer therapies
altitude training, mitochondria-strengthening
    benefits of, 133, 201

amalgam filling remediation, 6, 183–84

5-aminolevulinic acid (5ALA), 211

amygdala, 225–27

amygdalin (vitamin B$_{17}$), 162

anaerobic fermentation of carbohydrates, 128–130

anatomical man, 3, *ci1*

anti-infective therapies, 149–150

    See also infections

anti-inflammatory diet, 39–46

    cruciferous vegetables in, 34, 39–40

    fruits in, 42–45

    importance of, 154

    omega-3 fatty acids in, 41–42

    onion family in, 40–41

    supplements in, 45–46

Antonovsky, Aaron, 11

Aphorisms (Hippocrates), 168

apoptosis

    defined, 26

    energy needed for, 127

    goal of reviving, 128

    iodine role in, 188

    with local radio wave hyperthermia, 169–170

    mistletoe extracts for stimulation of, 198

arachidonic acid, 41, 56

Ardenne, Manfred von, 86–87, 171, 172

artemisinin, side effects of, 161

ashwagandha (*Withania somnifera*), 201

Aslan, Ana, 182

asparagus, selenium in, 69

aspartame, 112, 113

atorvastatin, cancer-inhibiting qualities of, 221, 222

ATP (adenosine triphosphate)

    energy production without oxygen, 128, 130

    energy production with oxygen, 127

    role in energy production, 126

autoimmune diseases

    chronic inflammation linked to, 147, 179

    immune system shifts and, 118

    iodine for, 189

    leaky gut linked to, 95

Ayurvedic medicine, 4

bacteria

    endosymbiont theory of mitochondria, 125

    inducing fever with, 170

    See also microbiome

bad-acid-forming foods, 75

    See also acid–base balance

balance, in health, 119–120, 155–58

    See also acid–base balance

base-forming foods

    fruits, 74*t*

    selecting, 76

    vegetables, 75*t*

bases, biochemistry of, 136–39

basic substance (extracellular matrix), 140

baths

    alkaline, 145

    hot, 35

    See also water therapies

beliefs, transforming unhealthy, 194–97

    See also inner life training; mindfulness training

berberine, blood glucose-regulating qualities,

    65, 197

berries

    in the anti-inflammatory diet, 43

    in the balanced and nutritious diet, 51–52

    vitamin C in, 66

Berry, Johann von, 3

Beschützt, bewahrt, geborgen (*Protected, Preserved,*

    Safe) (Francia), 84–85

best supportive care, as term, 224

beta-blockers, cancer-inhibiting qualities of, 222

beta-carotene, in cruciferous vegetables, 40

beverages

    in the acid–base balance-maintaining diet, 143

    detoxification role, 182

    good-acid-forming qualities, 76

    sugar in, 109

    See also water

binary representations, 7

biochemical processes

    acid-base balance and, 73, 136–39

    coherence in, 12

    complexity of, 5

biological anticancer agents

    hyperthermia treatments and, 172, 210

    insulin-potentiated therapy and, 166

    for restimulating lost apoptosis, 26

biophotonics, 24–25

biophotons, 23–29

Biophotons: The Light in Our Cells (Bischof), 27

biopsies and tissue examination, 214–16

bios (life force), 4

    See also chi/qi (vital force)

Bischof, Marco, 27
blood
    immune system and, 117–120
    intestinal and colon bleeding concerns, 219
    pH-balancing function of, 138–39
    pH value of, 137, 141
    titration with hydrochloric acid, 141
blood cell sedimentation rate (BSR) tests, 153
blood circulation
    acid–base balance benefits, 202
    PEMF benefits, 176
blood glucose regulation
    gut microbiome linked to, 94
    insulin-potentiated therapy and, 164–66
    low-carbohydrate diet benefits, 62–65
    natural remedies for, 197
    as one of the twelve vital fields, 9
blood tests
    for heavy metals, 183
    for inflammation parameters, 153, 179
    live blood analysis, 139, 176, ci2
body
    coherence in, 12
    physical vs. biochemical, 10
    soul vs., 10–11
Bohm, David, 4
Bohr, Niels, 237
Bojar, Hans, 216
boron, 186
Bosvene (boswellia preparation), 46
boswellic acids, 45–46
bradykinin, 89
brain
    childhood imprinting on, 100
    frontal lobe of, 225, 226
    gut–brain axis, 93
    holonomic model of, 4
    levels of consciousness, 120–21
    limbic system, 121, 217, 225, 227
    three parts of, 225
brainstem, 225
breast cancer
    chemotherapy effects, 107
    ginger for, 46
    iodine deficiency as risk factor for, 187
    iron deficiency as risk factor for, 186–87
    Japanese rates of, 16–17, 187
    preclinical observation of PEMF benefits, 176

screening examinations, 219
breast self-examination, 218
breast thermography, 219
breathing
    acid–base balance affected by, 143–44
    detoxification role, 182
    healthful approach to, 84–86
    in inner life training, 227–28
    oxygen from, 82–83
    See also oxygen
bromelain, for inflammation control, 44–45, 180
brush massage, 35, 182
Brussels sprouts, nutrients in, 40, 55
Budwig, Johanna, 28, 56
Budwig diet, 38, 56, 70
business of cancer treatment, 17–22
butyric acid, 59, 191
B vitamin group. See vitamin B group

cabbage family
    fermentation of, 47
    health benefits of, 34, 39–40
cachexia concerns, 65, 70
caesarean section, lack of contact with vaginal
    bacteria with, 92
cancer
    as disturbance of the vital force, xi
    as malignant variant of inflammation, 152
    most common types of, 16
    multifactorial etiology of, 5–8
    multiple levels of understanding, 237, ci8
    rising rates of, 15–17
Cancer as a Metabolic Disease (Seyfried), 129
cancer-associated fibroblasts, 83
cancer cells
    chlorophyll absorption by, 166–67
    chronic inflammation associated with, 151, 152
    circulating tumor cells, 215–16
    emission of noncoherent light, 26, 27
    heat shock protein formation, 168
    immune system shifts and, 116, 118, 121–22
    insulin receptors in, 165
    loss of adhesion molecules, 89
    lost apoptosis of, 26, 46, 128
    normal presence in the body, 150, 214
    sugar absorption by, 110
    See also tumors
cancer diagnosis. See diagnosis of cancer

cancer treatment. *See* treatment of cancer

cannabidiol (CBD), 200–201

cannabis terpenes, 200–201

carbohydrates

anaerobic fermentation of, 128–130

excessive consumption of, 129

in glycolysis, 126–27

in the healthy diet, 38

low-carbohydrate diet, 62–65

carbonated mineral water, 143

cardiovascular diseases

dietary recommendations for preventing, 41, 50, 54, 109, 132

mitochondrial damage linked to, 129

saturated fat consumption linked to, 53

sugar consumption linked to, 110, 112

cardiovascular exercise, 143–44, 203

L-carnitine, 73, 202

CAR T-cell therapy, 20

CBD (cannabidiol), 200–201

celecoxib

anti-inflammatory qualities, 152

cancer-inhibiting qualities of, 222

cells

biochemical reactions in, 5

complexity of, 5

light in, 23–29

See also cancer cells

Cells, Gels and the Engines of Life (Pollack), 80

cellular pathology, 3, 138

Cellular Pathology (Virchow), 3

cervical cancer

HPV infections linked to, 148

McLelland, Jane case, 221

screening examinations, 219

chakras, healing meditation based on, 233–34, *ci7*

chamomile, for gut health, 191, 204

chaos-coherence control circuits, 27

checkpoint inhibitors, 20, 168–69

chelation therapy, 183

chemosensitivity tests, 216

chemotherapy

grapefruit cautions, 44

hyperthermia with, 168

insulin-potentiated therapy and, 165–66

measurable effect on metastatic cancer survival, 107

mistletoe extracts with, 198, 199

probiotics during, 94

side effects, 166

vital mushroom extracts with, 199

as yang-intensive treatment, 209

chia seeds

for blood glucose regulation, 197

omega-3 fatty acids in, 55, 56

chi/qi (vital force)

connection with measurable energy, 28

defined, xi, 4

lack of physical measures for, 81

mitochondrial energy production correlated to, 127

chlamydial infections, ovarian cancer linked to, 148

chlorin e6 photosensitizer, 167, 210–11

chlorophyll, in photodynamic therapy, 166–67

Choleodoron (herbal remedy), 181

chromium, blood glucose-regulating qualities, 65, 197

chronic diseases

mitochondrial damage linked to, 129

stress linked to, 104

See also specific diseases

chronic infections

defined, 147

importance of finding and curing, 203–5

See also infections

chronic inflammation

autoimmune diseases linked to, 147

importance of finding and curing, 203–5

as silent inflammation, 150–54

transforming into acute inflammation, 151–52

chronic vs. acute acidosis, 135–36

chronic vs. acute stress, 99

See also stress

chymotrypsin, for inflammation control, 45, 180

cider vinegar, 65

cinnamon

for blood glucose regulation, 197

in the low-carbohydrate diet, 64

circulating tumor cells (CTCs), 215–16

citrate cycle, 127

citrus fruits, vitamin C in, 43, 66

Cleopatra (Egyptian queen), 173

clinical trials

alternatives to, 22

economic considerations, 18–19, 21, 132, 222

PEMF, 176–77

phases of, 19
    See also controlled, randomized studies
clove, Nf-Kappa-B inhibition by, 153
cocoa, in the low-carbohydrate diet, 64–65
coconut fat, as term, 54
coconut oil
    health benefits of, 54
    mitochondria-strengthening benefits of, 70–71
coenzyme Q10 (coQ10)
    acid–base balance benefits, 203
    mitochondria-strengthening benefits of, 72,
        132, 202
coffee
    enemas using, 35–36, 181
    Nf-Kappa-B inhibition by, 153
coffee charcoal, for gut health, 191, 204
cognitive trance, as term, 100
coherence, 8–14
    axes of resonance, 103
    biophotonics considerations, 25, 26
    chaos-coherence control circuits, 27
    healing meditations for, 123–25
    inner conflict in the immune system, 121–23
    interplay of physical and spiritual aspects, 10–14
    organic food considerations, 26
    as therapeutic concept for infections, 149–150
    twelve vital fields and, 9–10
coherent light, 25, 26, 27
colds, preventing, 35
cold training, mitochondria-strengthening
    benefits of, 133, 201
Coley, William B., 170
colon cancer
    bleeding concerns, 219
    chemotherapy effects, 107
    excessive iron as risk factor for, 186–87
    preclinical observation of PEMF benefits, 176
commensal bacteria, 90
    See also microbiome
complementary oncology, 159–177
    creating synergies, 159–163
    deacidification therapies, 142–45
    hyperthermia variations, 87, 151–52, 164,
        167–173, 182, 210
    insulin-potentiated therapy, 164–66, 210
    photodynamic therapy, 164, 166–67, 210–11
    principles of implementing vital field theory,
        163–65

pulsating electromagnetic frequency therapy,
    87–88, 173–77, 182, 190, 202, *ci2*
    working with conventional oncologists, 217–18
    yin and yang principle in, 209
complete response (CR), 212
connective tissue
    organ hypoxia effects on, 83
    pH value of, 137
conscious consciousness, as term, 121
consciousness
    distinction between self and not-self, 118–19
    frontal lobe of the brain and, 225
    healing meditations for, 123–25
    levels of, 120–21
    physically measurable changes in, 107
consciousness medicine, 120–23
controlled, randomized studies
    errors and misinterpretations in, 160
    requirements for, 18–19
    See also clinical trials
conventional cancer treatment
    doctrine of cancer treatment, 17–21
    guidelines in, 159
    interactions with naturopathic approaches,
        161–63, 217–18
    medicines as toxins, 32–34
    reductionist-materialist approach to, 3
    side effects from, 163–64
    view of health, 4–5
    yin and yang principle in, 209
coping strategies, 100–103
Corpus Hermeticum (ancient text), 2
costs. *See* economic considerations
CR (complete response), 212
C-reactive protein (CRP) blood tests, 153, 179
creatine, 72, 133
cruciferous vegetables
    in the anti-inflammatory diet, 39–40
    detoxification role, 34
CTCs (circulating tumor cells), 215–16
curcumin
    for inflammation control, 45, 180
    Nf-Kappa-B inhibition by, 152
cure, as term, 213, 214

dandelion extracts
    acid–base balance benefits, 203
    for detoxification, 181

dark field microscopy, 87–88, 139, 176, *ci2*

deacidification therapies, 142–45

Deadly Medicines and Organised Crime: How Big Pharma Has Corrupted Healthcare (Gøtzsche), 20

death
    after a full life, 237
    from overworking, 99
    preparing for, 223–24
    from stress, 105

decision making after diagnosis, 205–9

deep hyperthermia, 167–69

dental hygiene, importance of, 204

depression
    fever therapy benefits, 172
    gut microbiome imbalances linked to, 93
    mindfulness training benefits, 191

detoxification
    microbiome importance to, 92
    PEMF benefits, 176
    therapies for, 180–85
    vital field therapy approach to, 9, 30–36
    with whole-body hyperthermia, 172

detoxifying substances in food, 46–51

DHA (docosahexaenoic acid), 55, 56

diabetes
    blood glucose regulation-microbiome link and, 94
    controlling with diet, 43
    fruit consumption with, 42
    mitochondrial damage linked to, 129

diagnosis of cancer
    assessment criteria in, 212–13
    decision making after, 205–9
    examination methods, 213–14
    imaging methods, 110
    initial steps after, 216–18
    live blood analysis cautions, 139
    tissue examination, 214–16

diaphragm, 85

diaphragmatic breathing, 85

dichloroacetic acid, 132

diencephalon, 121

dietary fat. *See* fats

dietary fiber. *See* fiber

dietary recommendations
    acid–base balance-maintaining diet, 73–76, 74t, 75t, 142–43
    anti-inflammatory diet, 34, 39–46, 154

cardiovascular disease prevention, 41, 50, 54, 109, 132
    fats, 52–57
    gut health, 57–60
    immune system strengthening, 66–69
    infection control, 76–77
    low-carbohydrate diet, 62–65
    mitochondria-strengthening, 69–73
    nutrition principles, 36–38, 51–52
    stress-free eating, 60–62
    See also supplements

digestive enzymes
    anti-inflammatory qualities, 152
    pH value and, 137

digestive system. *See* gut health

dipyridamole, cancer-inhibiting qualities of, 221

disulfiram, cancer-inhibiting qualities of, 222

Dittrich-Opitz, Christian, 130

docosahexaenoic acid (DHA), 55, 56

doctrine of cancer treatment, 17–21
    See also conventional cancer treatment

do no harm principle, 163–64

dopamine, 93

dormant cancer cells, 26

doxycycline, cancer-inhibiting qualities of, 221, 222

drawing, as adjunct to fever therapy, 122, 173, *ci6*

D-ribose, 72

drinking water swirlers, 81–82, 189

drug cancer treatment. *See* pharmaceutical cancer treatment

duality principle, 3

economic considerations
    business of cancer treatment, 17–22
    clinical trials, 18–19, 21, 132, 222

ECS (endocannabinoid system), 200

"Effects of Psycho-Oncological Measures on the Survival Time of Cancer Patients" (study), 106–7

ego function, immune system and, 117–120

ego states (subpersonalities), 225

eicosapentaenoic acid (EPA), 55, 56

Einstein, Albert, 178

elderberry tea, for cold prevention, 35

electromagnetism, 174–75
    See also pulsating electromagnetic frequency (PEMF) therapy

electron potentials, 127

electrons, in redox reactions, 136, 137
electrosmog concerns, 174
Emerald Tablet (*Tabula Smaragdina*), 1–2
emotional well-being. *See* mental well-being
"Emotions as the Cause of Rapid and Sudden
   Death" (Yawger), 105
Empedocles, 2
endocannabinoid system (ECS), 200
endosymbiont theory of mitochondria, 125
endurance training
   acid–base balance benefits, 144, 203
   mitochondria-strengthening benefits, 134
enemas
   coffee, 35–36, 181
   for detoxification, 181
energy metabolism
   anaerobic fermentation of carbohydrates,
      128–130
   glycolysis, 126–27
   See also mitochondria
enzymes
   digestive, 137, 152
   pH value and, 137
   protein-splitting, 180
   vital mushrooms combined with, 199
eosinophils, 89
EPA (eicosapentaenoic acid), 55, 56
epigallocatechin gallate, 153
Equisetum arvense (horsetail) tea, 182
Erickson, Milton, 100, 124, 206
erythritol (sugar alcohol), 113–14, 116
essential fatty acids, 55–57
etiology of cancer
   biophotonics and, 25, 26
   lifestyle factors, 16–17
   multifactorial nature of, 5–8
   twelve vital fields in, 10
examinations
   for inflammation parameters, 153
   preventive, 204, 218–19
   types of, 213–14
exclusion zone (EZ) water, 79–82, *80*
exercise
   acid–base balance benefits, 76, 143–44, 203
   detoxifying effect of sweating, 181–82
   mitochondria-strengthening benefits, 201
   modern-day lack of, 129
   oxygen supply benefits, 189–190

exhaling, healthful approach to, 84–86
   See also breathing
extracellular matrix, 140

Farber, Sidney, 220
fasting. *See* intermittent fasting
fats, 52–57
   importance of, 52–53
   in the low-carbohydrate diet, 63–64
   mitochondria-strengthening benefits of, 69,
      70–71
   monounsaturated fatty acids, 54–55
   polyunsaturated fatty acids, 38, 55
   saturated fatty acids, 53–54, 70–71
Faust (Goethe), 117
fermentation of carbohydrates, anaerobic, 128–130
fermented foods, with lactic acid, 47–48, 59
ferritin blood tests, 153
fever therapy
   detoxifying effect of, 35
   drawing as adjunct to, 122, 173, *ci6*
   inflammation control with, 122
   with OMT, 87
   See also hyperthermia
fiber
   for blood glucose regulation, 197
   in cabbage, 40
   detoxifying effect of, 46–47
   for gut health, 58–59
   water-soluble vs. water-insoluble, 58
fibroblasts, cancer-associated, 83
field concept, 9–10
   See also twelve vital fields
fight-or-flight reactions, to cancer diagnosis, 217,
   225–26
filters, for water, 82
first, do no harm principle, 163–64
fish
   iodine in, 187
   in the low-carbohydrate diet, 63
   moral considerations in consumption of, 42
   omega-3 fatty acids in, 55, 63
fish oil supplements, 42, 56
flavonoids, 40, 44
flaxseed. *See* linseed (flaxseed)
fluid intake
   detoxification role, 182
   recommended amounts, 82

fluid intake (*continued*)

    See also beverages; water

fluorodeoxyglucose, in imaging studies, 110

folic acid

    acid–base balance benefits, 203

    immune system benefits, 68

food intolerances

    controlling with diet, 43

    fruit consumption with, 42

forgiveness, practicing, 192–93

Four Elements doctrine, 2–3

Four Humors Theory, 2–3

Francia, Luisa, 84–85

frankincense, 45–46

fraud concerns, 19–20, 162–63

free radicals

    alpha lipoic acid benefits, 132

    chronic inflammation associated with, 151

    mitochondria damaged by, 129–130

    resveratrol for, 132

    See also oxidative stress

freezing, as stress response, 226

freezing, of fruits and vegetables, 43

Friedman, Herbert, 23

Friesen, Claudia, 222

frontal lobe of the brain, 225, 226

frontal sinuses, controlling inflammation in, 204–5

fructose

    in fruits and vegetables, 42

    in honey, 114

    in onions, 41

fruits

    in the anti-inflammatory diet, 42–45

    in the balanced and nutritious diet, 51

    base-forming, 74t

    consuming peel of, 42, 43, 44, 58

    in green smoothies, 71

fruit vinegar, in the low-carbohydrate diet, 65

Full Catastrophe Living (Kabat-Zinn), 191

fuzzy logic and fuzzy sets, 6–7

GABA (gamma-aminobutyric acid), 93

Gaia (mythological figure), 235

gamma rays, 174

garlic

    in the anti-inflammatory diet, 40–41

    in the low-carbohydrate diet, 64

    sulfur in, 48

General Pathological Anatomy (Rokitansky), 3

general practitioner–centered care,

  in Germany, 33–34

genetic analysis

    of the microbiome, 190

    of tumors, 215

genistein, Nf-Kappa-B inhibition by, 152

German Cancer Research Center, 16

Germany

    general practitioner–centered care, 33–34

    mistletoe extract use, 198

    photodynamic therapy, 210

    revival of fever therapy, 171–72

    rising rates of cancer, 16

germ theory of disease, 149

Gerson, Max, 35–36, 181

Gesellschaft für Vitalpilzkunde e.V (Society for the Science of Vital Mushrooms), 199

ginger, in the anti-inflammatory diet, 46

ginkgo, Nf-Kappa-B inhibition by, 153

glucose

    absorption by cancer cells, 110

    anaerobic fermentation of, 128–130

    in fruits and vegetables, 42

    glycolysis of, 126–27

    in honey, 114

    See also sugar

glucose tolerance factor (GTF), 197

glucosinolates, 34, 39, 40, 48

glycocalyx, 138

goal setting for change, 107–8

Goethe, Johann Wolfgang von, 29, 82, 117, 127, 158

good-acid-forming foods, 75

    See also acid–base balance

good life with cancer, 236–38, *ci8*

Gøtzsche, Peter Christian, 19–20

gout, from uric acid, 32

grapefruit, caution in consumption of, 44

Great Hymn to the Aton (Akhenaten), 28

green leafy vegetables

    base-forming vegetables, 75t

    in green smoothies, 71

    in the low-carbohydrate diet, 63

green smoothies, 70, 71

guidelines, for conventional cancer treatment, 159

Gurwitsch, Alexander, 23–24, 28

gut–brain axis, 93

gut health, 89–96
    blood glucose regulation and, 94
    dietary recommendations for, 57–60
    examination of intestinal flora and immunol-
        ogy, 153
    gut–brain axis, 93
    importance of monitoring, 204
    leaky gut syndrome, 94–96, 184
    microbiome and, 57, 90–94, 190, 204
    as one of the twelve vital fields, 9
    overview, 89–90
    therapies for, 190–91
gynecological cancers, mistletoe extracts for, 198
gynecological examinations, importance of, 204

haem oxygenase-1, 89
Hazuda, Helen, 111
healing clay, for blood glucose regulation, 197
healing crises, with fever, 122
healing meditations, 123–25, 229–235, ci7
healing trances, 124
health
    as balance between toxification and
        detoxification, 30–31
    conventional medicine view of, 4–5
    oscillating balance in, 119–120
healthy eating. See nutrition
heat shock proteins, 168
heat therapy. See hyperthermia
heavy metals, detoxification from, 183–84
Heckel, Martin, 171, 172
Helicobacter pylori infections, 91, 148
hepatitis infections, 148
Heraclitus, 155
hermeticism, role in the holistic principle, 2, 3
hexagonal structure of exclusion zone water,
    80–81, 80
highly sensitive C-reactive protein (hsCRP)
    blood tests, 179
Hippocrates, 2, 8, 89, 163, 168, 173
holistic principle, 1–14
    coherence and health, 8–14
    complexity and unambiguity, 5–8
    defined, 1
    history of, 1–5
    See also twelve vital fields
holonomic brain model, 4
hólons, hierarchy of, 1

homeostasis, 10, 155
    See also balance, in health
honey
    consumption of, 109
    multiple uses of, 114–15, 116
hormesis principle, 88, 152
horsetail (Equisetum arvense) tea, 182
HPA axis (hypothalamic-pituitary-adrenal axis),
    97, 98
HPV (human papilloma virus) infections, 148
hydrochloric acid, titration of blood using, 141
hydrogen, as reducing agent, 137
hydrogenated fats, avoiding, 53, 54
hyperacidity
    chronic vs. acute acidosis, 135–36
    health problems with, 138, 139
    inflammation linked to, 140, 151
    measurement methods, 141–42
hyperthermia, 167–173
    in complementary oncology, 164
    deep, 167–69
    local application of, 169–170, 210
    mental healing and, 172–73
    in oxygen multistep therapy, 87
    transforming chronic inflammation into acute
        with, 151–52
    whole-body, 170–72, 182
    See also fever therapy
hypnotherapy, 100, 105, 124
hypochondrium, as term, 94–95
hypothalamic-pituitary-adrenal axis (HPA axis),
    97, 98
hypoxia training, 131, 133, 201

IHHT (intermittent hypoxia–hyperoxia therapy),
    131, 133, 201
immune system, 116–125
    consciousness medicine for, 120–23
    dietary recommendations for strengthening,
        66–69
    ego function and, 117–120
    healing meditations for, 123–25
    immune cell types, 116–17
    inflammation associated with, 146–47, 151
    influence of feelings on, 156
    inner conflict in, 121–23
    microbiome importance to, 92
    Nf-Kappa-B role in, 152–53

immune system (*continued*)
  as one of the twelve vital fields, 9
  optimization strategies, 198–201
  PEMF benefits, 176
  psychoneuroimmunology field, 98–99, 106–7,
    120–23, 156
immunotherapy
  costs of, 20
  hyperthermia with, 168–69
incompetence-compensation-competence, 108
Indian sleeping berry (*Withania somnifera*), 201
individualized medicine, 160, 161
induction, absorption of pulsating e
  lectromagnetic frequency energy by, 175
infants
  contact with bacterial colonization of the
    birth canal, 91–92
  honey cautions, 115
infection control
  nutrition for, 76–77
  as one of the twelve vital fields, 9, 145–150
infections
  causes and symptoms of, 145–49
  chronic inflammation associated with, 150–54
  immune system shift caused by, 117
  increased risk of cancer from, 147–48
  intracellular, 148
  microbe–host relationships vs., 149
  types of, 147
inflammation
  acid-base balance importance in, 140
  chronic, 147, 150–54, 203–5
  damage from, 39
  immune system interactions with, 116, 117,
    146–47
  increased uptake of sugar with, 110
  from leaky gut, 95
  as self-force, 120
  symptoms of, 146
inflammation control
  dietary recommendations for, 34, 39–46, 154
  fever therapy benefits, 122
  as one of the twelve vital fields, 9
  resveratrol for, 132
  therapies for, 179–180
inflammatory foci, as term, 153
infrared whole-body hyperthermia therapy,
  171–72, 190

infusion therapy
  local radio wave hyperthermia with, 170
  whole-body hyperthermia with, 172
inhalation therapy. *See* intermittent hypoxia–
  hyperoxia therapy (IHHT)
inner life training, 224–29, *ci7*
  See also mindfulness training
Institute for Applied Epistemology and Medical
  Methodology (Witten-Herdecke University), 22
insulin
  blood glucose regulation and, 197
  receptors in cancer cells, 165
insulin-potentiation therapy (IPT), 164–66, 210
insulin sensitivity, intermittent fasting benefits, 134
integrative medicine, synergies in, 159–163, 164
  See also complementary oncology
intermittent fasting
  for blood glucose regulation, 197
  mitochondria-strengthening benefits of, 70, 134
intermittent hypoxia–hyperoxia therapy (IHHT),
  131, 133, 201
interventional radiology treatments, 211
intestinal cleansing powders, 47, 59
intestinal flora and immunology, examination
  of, 153
intestinal health. *See* gut health
intestines
  bleeding concerns, 219
  detoxification via, 181
  mucosal barrier of, 95
intolerances. *See* food intolerances
intracellular infections, 148
intravenous oxyvenation therapy (IOT), 88–89
inulin, for blood glucose regulation, 197
iodine
  importance of, 187, 188–89
  supplementation with, 186, 187–88
IOT (intravenous oxyvenation therapy), 88–89
IPT (insulin-potentiation therapy), 164–66, 210
iron
  acid–base balance benefits, 203
  immune system benefits, 68–69
  in legumes, 49
  supplementation with, 186–87
isomalt (sugar alcohol), 113–14

Japan
  breast cancer rates, 16–17

death from overworking, 99
meal habits, 61

Kabat-Zinn, Jon, 103, 191
kaempferol
    in cruciferous vegetables, 40
    detoxifying effect of, 50
    dosage concerns, 50
karoshi (death from overworking), 99
ketogenic diet
    mitochondria strengthening benefits of, 72, 134
    sugar alcohols for, 113
Keupp, Heiner, 12–13
kidneys, detoxification role, 34, 182
Kneipp, Sebastian, 145
Kneipp applications
    acid–base balance benefits, 144–45, 202
    mitochondria-strengthening benefits,
        144–45, 201
Know, Lee, 73
knowledge-based vs. evidence-based medicine, 22
Koch, Robert, 149
Krauss, Werner, 174
Kreutzer, Frank, 89
Küchler, Thomas, 106–7

lactic acid
    formation during anaerobic fermentation of
        carbohydrates, 128, 129
    production in tumors, 83, 141
lactic acid bacteria, for gut health, 47–48, 59–60
Lao Tse, 102
laser light
    coherence of, 25
    in photodynamic therapy, 166, 167, 210–11
latent infections, 147
    See also infections
lauric acid, 70–71
L-carnitine, 73, 202
leaky gut syndrome, 94–96, 184
Lechner, Fritz, 174
legumes
    detoxifying effect of, 49
    good-acid-forming qualities, 75
    in the low-carbohydrate diet, 63
    selenium in, 69
lemon, in the anti-inflammatory diet, 43–44
letting go, in mindfulness training, 192

leukemia treatment, 219–220
life force. See chi/qi (vital force)
light
    in cells, 23–29
    healing meditations for, 231, 235, ci7
    laser light, 25, 166, 167, 210–11
limbic system, 121, 217, 225, 227
Limbourg brothers, 2, ci1
limonoids, 43
linoleic acid, 56
linseed (flaxseed)
    for blood glucose regulation, 197
    fiber in, 58, 197
    healthy fats in, 55, 56
Lipton, Bruce, 156
live blood analysis, 139, 176, ci2
liver
    acid–base balance optimization and, 203
    alcohol breakdown in, 32
    coffee enemas for, 36
    detoxification role, 34
    natural remedies for detoxifying, 181
    pathological detoxification of, 31
liver-activating substances, 34
liver cancer
    hepatitis infections linked to, 148
    observed PEMF benefits, 176, 177
    transarterial chemoembolization for, 211
living with cancer, 100–103, 236–38, ci8
local deep hyperthermia, 167–69
local radio wave hyperthermia, 169–170, 210
London Care Oncology Clinic, 222
Longo, Valter, 70
love, healing meditation for, 232
low-carbohydrate diet, 62–65
Lugol's solution, 188
lung cancer
    chemotherapy effects, 107
    transarterial chemoembolization for, 211
lungs, 85
Luzbetak, Martin, 216

macrophages, 116–17, 120
magnesium
    acid–base balance benefits, 203
    mitochondria-strengthening benefits, 72
    in oxygen multistep therapy, 87
    supplementation with, 186

magnetic therapy. *See* pulsating electromagnetic frequency (PEMF) therapy

magnetism, 174–75

  See also pulsating electromagnetic frequency (PEMF) therapy

malignancy, defined, 140

malignant melanoma, preclinical observation of PEMF benefits, 176

mammary glands, importance of iodine to, 187, 188

manganese, acid–base balance benefits, 203

mannitol (sugar alcohol), 114

Marquard, Odo, 108

McLelland, Jane, 221

mealtimes, stress-free, 60–62

mebendazole, cancer-inhibiting qualities of, 221, 222

medical professionals. *See* practitioners

meditations, healing, 123–25, 229–235, *ci7*

medium-chain triglycerides (MCTs), 54, 70–71

mental well-being

  acid–base balance affected by, 144

  coherence in the mind and, 11, 12

  defined, 11

  distinction between self and not-self, 118–19

  fever therapy benefits, 172–73

  professional support for, 218

  resolution of inner conflict benefits, 122–23

  role of imagination in healing, 105

  transforming unhealthy beliefs, 194–97

  See also inner life training; mindfulness training

mercury, in amalgam fillings, 183

Messner, Franz Anton, 173

metastasis

  biopsy concerns, 214–15

  goal of dormant cancer for, 26

  intravenous oxyvenation therapy benefits, 89

  Nf-Kappa-B role in, 152

metformin, cancer-inhibiting qualities of, 220, 221, 222

methadone, cancer-inhibiting qualities of, 222

methylsulfonylmethane (MSM)

  anti-inflammatory qualities, 49

  detoxifying effect of, 34, 181, 183

microbe–host relationships, as term, 149

  See also infections

microbiome

  blood glucose regulation linked to, 94

  genetic analysis of, 190

gut health and, 57, 90–94, 204

  See also gut health

microcirculation therapies, 86–89

microcosm-macrocosm relationship, 77

micronutrients

  acid–base balance benefits, 203

  detoxifying effects, 50–51

  in green smoothies, 71

midbrain, 225

  See also brain

milk thistle

  acid–base balance benefits, 203

  detoxifying effect of, 50, 181

mindfulness training

  clear, conscious thinking and, 121

  living a good life with cancer, 236–37

  for stress reduction, 103–7, 191–93

  See also inner life training

minerals

  adsorption of toxins, 184–85

  in legumes, 49

  See also specific minerals

mineral water, carbonated, 143

mistletoe extracts, for immune system optimization, 198–99

mitochondria, 125–134

  aging and, 130–34

  anaerobic fermentation of carbohydrates, 128–130

  dietary recommendations for strengthening, 69–73

  need for more research on, 28

  as one of the twelve vital fields, 9

  structure and function of, 125–28, *126*

  treatments and supplements for strengthening, 131–34, 201–2

Mitochondria and the Future of Medicine (Know), 73

Mitochondria: More Life Energy Due to Healthy Cellular Power Plants (Dittrich-Opitz), 130

mitogenetic radiation, 24

mitosis, influence of biophotons on, 24

Modern Acid-Base Medicine (van Limburg Stirum), 141

monounsaturated fatty acids, 54–55

morphogenetic fields, 27, 81

mouth and jaw, examination of, 153

MSM (methylsulfonylmethane)

  anti-inflammatory qualities, 49

  detoxifying effect of, 34, 181, 183

mucosal barrier, intestinal, 95
mushrooms
    in the balanced and nutritious diet, 52
    proteases in, 180
    vital mushroom extracts, 199
myrosinase, in cabbage, 40
myrrh, for gut health, 191, 204

nasal sinuses, controlling inflammation in, 204–5
"Nature: Fragment f rom the Journal of Tiefurt"
    (Goethe), 127
naturopathy
    interactions with conventional medicine,
        161–63
    synergies in, 159–161
    treatment of disturbed acid–base balance, 135
    vital force used by, xi
    yin principle in, 209
    See also complementary oncology
Nauts, Helen Coley, 170
NED (no evidence of disease), 214
neurodegenerative diseases, mitochondrial
    damage linked to, 129
Nf-Kappa-B, 152–53
no evidence of disease (NED), 214
nonjudgmental thinking, in mindfulness
    training, 191
nononcological drug treatment, 220–23
nonstriving, in mindfulness training, 192
Novalis (poet), 223
Now (Tolle), 101–2
nutrition
    as one of the twelve vital fields, 9
    principles of, 36–38, 51–52
    supplements for nutritional deficiencies,
        185–89, 186t
    See also dietary recommendations

obesity
    blood glucose regulation-microbiome link
        and, 94
    mitochondrial damage linked to, 129
    sugar substitutes linked to, 111–12
oily fish, in the low-carbohydrate diet, 63
    See also fish
omega-3 fatty acids
    anti-inflammatory qualities, 41–42, 152, 180
    ratio to omega-6 fatty acids, 57

role in nutrition, 55–56
    supplementation with, 186
omega-6 fatty acids
    potentially inflammatory qualities, 41, 42, 57
    ratio to omega-3 fatty acids, 57
    role in nutrition, 56–57
OMT (oxygen multistep therapy), 86–87
oncologists, burnout in, 96
oncology. See complementary oncology;
    conventional cancer treatment
onion family
    in the anti-inflammatory diet, 40–41
    sulfur in, 48
"On the Aesthetic Education of Man" (Schiller),
    156–57
oregano, Nf-Kappa-B inhibition by, 153
organically developed toxins, 32
organic food
    base-forming foods, 76
    light emission from, 25–26
orthomolecular medicine
    mitochondria-strengthening benefits of, 131, 202
    yin principle in, 209
outside-the-box cancer therapies, 178–235
    acid–base balance optimization, 202–3
    assessment criteria for diagnosis and
        treatment, 212–19
    decision making after diagnosis, 205–9
    detoxification, 180–85
    fresh water, 189
    healing meditations, 229–235
    immune system optimization, 198–201
    infection control, 203–5
    inflammation control, 179–180
    inner life training, 224–29
    insulin and blood sugar regulation, 197
    intestinal remediation, 190–91
    leukemia treatment, 219–220
    mindfulness training, 191–93
    mitochondria medicine, 201–2
    nononcological drug treatment, 220–23
    overview, 178–79
    oxygen supply, 189–190
    palliative care, 223–24
    supplements, 185–89, 186t
    transformation of unhealthy beliefs, 194–97
    tumor-killing treatment methods, 209–12
    See also complementary oncology

ovarian cancer
  chlamydial infections linked to, 148
  oncobiome for, 94
overacidification. *See* hyperacidity
oxidative stress
  coenzyme Q10 for, 132
  detoxifying food substances for, 50
  intermittent fasting for, 134
  mitochondria damaged by, 129–130
  selenium for, 69
  See also free radicals
oxygen, 82–89
  acid–base balance optimization and, 202
  cancer growth and, 82–86
  in glycolysis, 127
  increased uptake with PEMF, 175, 176
  as one of the twelve vital fields, 9
  as oxidizing agent, 137
  therapies with, 86–89, 172, 189–190, 202
oxygen deficiencies
  chronic inflammation associated with, 151
  immune system shift caused by, 116, 117
oxygen multistep therapy (OMT), 86–87
oxyvenation therapy, intravenous (IOT), 88–89
ozone therapy, 145, 202

pain
  affirmations for, 229
  with inflammation, 146
  inner life training affirmations for, 229
  methadone for, 222
  PEMF for, 175, 177
  THC for, 200–201
palliative care, 223–24
pancreatin, for inflammation control, 180
papain, for inflammation control, 44–45, 180
Paracelsus, 30, 152, 173
para oxygenase-1, 89
parasite infections, controlling, 204
Parmenides, 168
partial response (PR), 213
Pasteur, Louis, 149
pathological tissue examination, 214–16
patience, in mindfulness training, 192
Pauling, Linus, 131
PD (progressive disease), 213
PDT (photodynamic therapy), 164, 166–67, 210–11
pectin, 42, 58

peel of fruits, 42, 43, 44, 58
PEMF therapy. *See* pulsating electromagnetic
  frequency (PEMF) therapy
peracute infections, 147
  See also infections
Perez Garcia, Donato, Jr., 165
Perez Garcia, Donato, Sr., 165
PET (positron emission tomography), 110
PET-CT (positron emission tomography and
  computer tomography), 110, 214
pH
  defined, 137
  of the human body, 73, 137
  measurement methods, 141–42
pharmaceutical cancer treatment
  costs of, 20
  efficacy of, 19
  See also chemotherapy; conventional
  cancer treatment
photodynamic therapy (PDT), 164, 166–67, 210–11
photomultipliers, 24
photon emission, ultraweak, 24
photons, 23–24
  See also biophotons
photosensitizers, 167, 210–11
physical activity. *See* exercise
physicians. *See* practitioners
phytochemicals
  in cabbage, 34, 39, 40
  detoxifying effect of, 50
pineapple, in the anti-inflammatory diet, 44
Pischinger, Alfred, 138, 140
Pollack, Gerald H., 79, 80
polyphenols
  in cocoa, 64
  detoxifying effect of, 50
  in red wine, 133
polysaccharides, in vital mushrooms, 199
polyunsaturated fatty acids, 38, 55
Popp, Fritz-Albert, 24, 25, 26, 27, 28
pork, avoiding, 41
potatoes, boiled in their skins, 59
potentiation effect, 168
PQQ (pyrroloquinoline quinone), 72, 132, 202
PR (partial response), 213
practitioners
  consulting with, 178–79, 185–86, 205–6, 207, 223
  first, do no harm principle, 163–64

general practitioner–centered care, in
Germany, 33–34
palliative care decisions, 223–24
prana (vital force)
connection with measurable energy, 28
defined, xi, 4
lack of physical measures for, 81
mitochondrial energy production correlated
to, 127
prebiotics, 191, 204
prevalence of cancer, 15–17
preventive examinations, importance of,
204, 218–19
Pribram, Karl H., 4
probiotics
with anti-infective therapies, 150
during chemotherapy, 94
for gut health, 47–48, 60, 191, 204
procaine-base infusions, 182–83, 203
programmed cell death-1 receptors (PD-1
receptors), 20
progressive disease (PD), 213
prostacyclin, 89
prostate cancer
chemotherapy effects, 107
rates in China, 17
screening examinations, 219
prostate examinations, importance of, 204
proteases
for inflammation control, 180
vital mushrooms combined with, 199
Protected, Preserved, Safe (Beschützt, bewahrt,
geborgen) (Francia), 84–85
protein precipitations, between blood cells, 139
protein-splitting enzymes, 180
proton pump inhibitors, 140
protons
in acid-base reactions, 136, 137, 140
in glycolysis, 127
psyche, as term, 11
psychological health. See mental well-being
psychoneuroimmunology (PNI)
consciousness medicine and, 120–23
emergence of field, 98–99
influence of feelings on the immune system, 156
research on benefits of psychotherapeutic
support, 106–7
psycho-oncology, 11, 100, 106–8

psyllium
for blood glucose regulation, 197
for gut health, 46, 58, 59
pulsating electromagnetic frequency
(PEMF) therapy
acid–base balance benefits, 202
dark field microscopy before and after, ci2
detoxification benefits, 182
mitochondria-strengthening benefits, 202
oxygen supply benefits, 87–88, 190
role in complementary oncology, 173–77
purple potatoes, cancer-fighting effects of, 59
pyretotherapy. See fever therapy
pyrroloquinoline quinone (PQQ), 72, 132, 202
pyruvate (pyruvic acid), 127, 128

qi (vital force). See chi/qi (vital force)
quercetin
in cruciferous vegetables, 40
detoxifying effect of, 50
dosage concerns, 50
Nf-Kappa-B inhibition by, 152
in the onion family, 40, 41

radiation therapy
evaluation of, 207
gamma rays used in, 174
grapefruit cautions, 44
hyperthermia with, 168
local radio wave hyperthermia with, 170
Radical Forgiveness (Tipping), 192–93
Radical Remission: Surviving Cancer Against All
Odds (Turner), 100, 157, 190
radiofrequency ablation, 211
radioligand therapy, 211–12
radiology treatments, interventional, 211
radio wave hyperthermia, local, 169–170, 210
rates of cancer, rising, 15–17
RECIST (response evaluation criteria in solid
tumors) criteria, 212–13
red blood cells
iron needed for, 49, 68
rouleaux formation phenomenon, 87–88, 139
sedimentation rate testing, 153
red meat, limiting consumption of, 41, 186–87
redox reactions, 136–37
reductionist-materialist approach to medicine, 3
See also conventional cancer treatment

red wine, resveratrol in, 132–33
"Reflexive Social Psychology" (Keupp), 12–13
Regelsberger, Helmut, 88–89
regional deep hyperthermia, 167–69
  See also hyperthermia
relapsing infections, 147
  See also infections
reptilian brain, as term, 225, 226
research on cancer
  clinical trials, 18–19, 21, 22, 132, 176–77, 222
  controlled, randomized studies, 18–19, 160
  conventional medicine doctrine, 17–21
  costs of, 18–19
  knowledge-based vs. evidence-based
    medicine, 22
  self-contained system of medical research, 21–22
  statistical analysis of, 207–9
Resonance: A Sociology of Modernity (Resonanz—
  eine Soziologie der Moderne) (Rosa), 103
resonance axes of health, 103
resonance principle, 29
respiratory chain, 126
response evaluation criteria in solid tumors
  (RECIST) criteria, 212–13
rest needs, 62
resveratrol
  anti-inflammatory qualities, 152
  detoxifying effect of, 50
  mitochondria-strengthening benefits of,
    72, 132–33
reverse osmosis water treatment systems, 189
Rhodiola rosea, 201
D-ribose, 72
Rokitansky, Karl von, 3
root-treated teeth and gums, 204
Rosa, Hartmut, 101, 103
rouleaux formation phenomenon, 87–88, 139, ci2

saccharin, metabolic diseases linked to, 112, 113
safe feelings, healing meditation for, 230
saliva, pH of, 141
salutogenesis model, 11
saturated fatty acids
  in the balanced and nutritious diet, 53–54
  mitochondria-strengthening benefits of, 70–71
sauerkraut, probiotics in, 47, 48
saunas, detoxification through, 181–82, 190
Schamhart, Dennis, 27

Schiller, Friedrich, 156–57
Schmid, Gary Bruno, 105
sclerotherapy with radiofrequency, 211
screening programs, 219
SD (stable disease), 213
sea buckthorn, vitamin C in, 44
search reflex, 121
seasonal foods, 51
selenium
  detoxifying effect of, 50, 181
  immune system benefits, 69
  supplementation with, 186
self-contained system of medical research, 21–22
Self-Healing by Imagination (Schmid), 105
Selye, Hans, 96–97
semiconscious consciousness, 121
serotonin, gut microbiome linked to, 93, 94
seven chakras, healing meditation based on,
  233–34, ci7
Seyfried, Thomas N., 129
Sheldrake, Rupert, 27, 81
6-shogaol, 46
Siberian ginseng, 201
side effects
  from conventional cancer treatment,
    163–64, 221
  from naturopathic treatments, 161
  from nononcological drugs, 221, 223
  treatment decision making and, 207, 223
significant correlation, defined, 208
sildenafil (Viagra), cancer-inhibiting qualities of, 222
silymarin, detoxifying effect of, 50, 181
Simonton, Oscar Carl, 108, 194, 205
sinuses, controlling inflammation in, 204–5
skin, detoxification via, 181–82
skin cancer, screening examinations, 219
sleep needs, 62
Smith, Edwin, 167
smoothies, green, 70, 71
social factors, in stress, 97–98, 101
Society for the Science of Vital Mushrooms
  (Gesellschaft für Vitalpilzkunde e.V), 199
sodium cyclamate (sugar substitute), 113
sodium hydrogen carbonate, in procaine-base
  infusions, 183
Soffritti, Morando, 112
Sönnichsen, Andreas, 33
sorbitol (sugar alcohol), 114

sorites paradox, 7

soul, body and spirit vs., 10–11

   See also mental well-being

soy, fermented, good-acid-forming qualities, 76

sparkling water, 143

   See also water

sports. *See* exercise

stable disease (SD), 213

standardized uptake values (SUVs), 110

state of health, 10, 30, 216

statistical analysis of medical studies, 207–9

statistically significant effects, defined, 208

Steiner, Rudolf, 198

stevia and steviol glycosides, 114, 116

stomach cancer

   Helicobacter pylori infections linked to, 91, 148

   proton pump inhibitors for, 140

stress, 96–108

   coping with cancer, 100–103

   fight-or-flight reactions, 217, 225–26

   goal setting for change, 107–8

   mindfulness against, 103–7

   origins of, 96–100, 98

   triggers for, 104–5

   See also oxidative stress

stress-free eating, 60–62

stress hormones, 97, 226

stress management

   inner life training, 224–29, ci7

   mindfulness training, 103–7, 121, 191–93, 236–37

   as one of the twelve vital fields, 9

   transforming unhealthy beliefs, 194–97

Stress och den nya ohälsan (*Stress and the New Unhealthiness*) (Währborg), 96

Stress Reduction Clinic (University of Massachusetts), 103

structured water (EZ water), 79–82, 80

sub-acute infections, 147

   See also infections

subconscious level of consciousness, 120–21

subpersonalities (ego states), 225

sucralose, metabolic diseases linked to, 112, 113

sucrose, in honey, 109

sugar

   dangers of, 108–11

   substitutes for, 111–16

sugar alcohols, 113–14, 116

sugar crises, 165–66

sulfur, detoxifying effect of, 34, 48–49, 183

The Sun (Friedman), 23

sun, significance to life, 23

   See also light

supplements

   in the anti-inflammatory diet, 45–46

   for balanced insulin levels, 65

   choosing in consultation with practitioners, 178–79

   for detoxification, 50–51

   fiber, 46, 59

   for immune system strengthening, 66–69

   mitochondria-strengthening benefits of, 71–73, 131–33

   for nutritional deficiencies, 185–89, 186t

   sulfur, 34, 49

SUVs (standardized uptake values), 110

Swa-Dhisthana (second chakra), 108

Swanton, Charles, 19

sweating, detoxification through, 34, 35, 181–82

sweeteners (sugar substitutes), 111–13

   See also sugar

swirling devices, for structured water, 81–82, 189

symbiosis therapy, 204

symbiotic bacteria, balance and specialization in, 90–91

syncytia, loss of, 27, 130

Tabula Smaragdina (Emerald Tablet), 1–2

TACE (transarterial chemoembolization), 211

Tantric Buddhism, chakras in, 233, ci7

Tao Te Ching (Lao Tse), 102

THC (tetrahydrocannabinol), 200–201

Theory of the Four Humors, 2–3

therapy for cancer. *See* treatment of cancer

thermogenesis, mitochondria-strengthening benefits of, 133

thermography, breast, 219

thiamine

   in legumes, 49

   in oxygen multistep therapy, 87

thyme, Nf-Kappa-B inhibition by, 153

thyroid hormones, iodine in, 188

Tipping, Colin, 192–93

tocotrienols, Nf-Kappa-B inhibition by, 153

Tolle, Eckhart, 101–2

Tomasetti, Cristian, 7–8

tooth roots, inflamed, 153, 204

toxins
  environmental, 31
  free radicals from, 130
  heavy metals, 183–84
  immune system shift caused by, 117
  medicines as, 32–34
  organically developed, 32
  See also detoxification
Traditional Chinese Medicine (TCM), 4
transarterial chemoembolization (TACE), 211
trans fats, avoiding, 53
treatment of cancer
  business of, 17–22
  evaluation of, 206–9, 213–14
  multifactorial nature of, 5–6
  twelve vital fields in, 9
  See also complementary oncology;
    conventional cancer treatment
Les Très Riches Heures du Duc de Berry (Berry), 2–3, ci1
Trismegistos, Hermes, 1–2
trust, in mindfulness training, 192
trypsin, for inflammation control, 45, 180
tumors
  acid–base imbalance between inner and outer
    milieu, 140
  biopsies of, 214–16
  essence of, 120
  heterogeneity of tissue, 215
  hyperthermia effects on, 168–69
  immune system shift toward, 116, 120
  lactic acid production by, 141
  markers for, 215
  special tumor-killing treatment methods, 209–12
  Vogelstein and Tomasetti study, 7–8
  See also cancer cells
turmeric, anti-inflammatory qualities, 152, 153, 180
Turner, Kelly, 100, 157, 190
twelve vital fields, 30–154
  acid–base balance importance, 9, 135–36, 140
  acid–base balance-maintaining diet, 73–76,
    74t, 75t
  acid–base biochemistry, 136–39, 141–42
  anaerobic fermentation of carbohydrates,
    128–130
  anti-inflammatory diet, 34, 39–46, 154
  balance in, 155–58, ci3, ci4, ci5
  blood glucose regulation, 9, 62–65, 94,
    164–66, 197

coherence and, 9–10, 11
complementary deacidification therapies,
  142–45
complementary oncology guided by, 163–65
coping with cancer, 100–103
detoxification of the organism, 9, 30–36, 92,
  172, 176, 180–85
detoxifying substances in food, 46–51
ego function and the immune system, 117–120
fat types and needs, 52–57, 63–64, 69, 70–71
goal setting for change, 107–8
gut health, 9, 57–60, 89–96, 153, 184, 190–91, 204
healing meditations, 123–25, 229–235, ci7
immune cell transformations, 116–17
immune system strengthening, 9, 66–69
infection control, 9, 76–77, 145–150
inflammation control, 9, 34, 39–46, 132,
  150–54, 179–180
interrelationships among, 77
mindfulness training, 103–7, 121, 191–93,
  236–37
mitochondrial health, 9, 69–73, 130–34
mitochondrial structure and function,
  125–28, 126
nutrition principles, 9, 36–38, 51–52
overview, 8–10
oxygen needs, 9, 82–89
psychoneuroimmunology and, 120–23
sources of stress, 96–100, 98
stress-free eating, 60–62
stress management, 9, 191–97, 224–29
sugar dangers, 108–16
systemic thinking behind, 38
water needs, 9, 52, 78–82, 80

ultraweak photon emission, 24
unprejudiced thinking, in mindfulness training, 192
Uranos (mythological figure), 235
uric acid, gout from, 32
urine, pH of, 141

vaginal bacteria, newborn contact with, 91–92
vaginal seeding, 92
van Limburg Stirum, Johan, 141
vegetables
  in the balanced and nutritious diet, 51
  base-forming, 75t
  cruciferous, 34, 39–40

green leafy, 63, 71, 75t
  in the low-carbohydrate diet, 63
Viagra (sildenafil), cancer-inhibiting
  qualities of, 222
Virchow, Rudolf, 3, 138
vis vitalis (life force), 4
  See also chi/qi (vital force)
vital fields, 27, 149
  See also twelve vital fields
vital force. See chi/qi (vital force)
vital mushroom extracts, 199
vitamin B₁. See thiamine
vitamin B₁₂, 68
vitamin B₁₇ (amygdalin), 162
vitamin B group
  acid–base balance benefits, 203
  in cruciferous vegetables, 40
  immune system benefits, 68
  mitochondria-strengthening benefits, 72
vitamin C
  in citrus fruits, 43, 44
  costs of, 20
  in cruciferous vegetables, 40
  detoxifying effect of, 50
  fraudulent claims about, 162
  immune system benefits, 66–67
  lack of insurance coverage for, 19, 21
  in oxygen multistep therapy, 87
  in sea buckthorn, 44
  supplementation with, 186
  whole-body hyperthermia with, 172
vitamin D
  deficiency in, 185, 186t
  immune system benefits, 67
  supplementation with, 186
vitamin K, 40
Vogelstein, Bert, 7–8
von Ardenne, Manfred, 86–87, 171, 172

Währborg, Peter, 96
walnuts, Nf-Kappa-B inhibition by, 153
Warburg, Otto, 86, 129, 171
warmth and light, healing meditation for, 231
water
  acid–base balance affected by, 145
  chemical formulas for, 78, 80
  daily needs, 78

exclusion zone (EZ) water, 79–82, 80
  for fiber digestion, 58
  importance to health, 52, 78–81, 189
  as one of the twelve vital fields, 9
  sparkling, 143
  treatment of, 81–82, 189
Water: Much More Than H₂O (Pollack), 79
water-soluble vs. water-insoluble fiber, 58
water therapies
  baths, 35, 145
  cold training, 133, 201
  Kneipp applications, 144–45, 201, 202
Wegman, Ita, 198
"What Is Cognition-Based Medicine" (article), 22
white blood cells
  CAR T-cell therapy, 20
  immune system role of, 118
whole-body hyperthermia, 170–72, 182
whole-grain foods
  fiber in, 58
  good-acid-forming qualities, 75–76
  in the low-carbohydrate diet, 63
Withania somnifera (Indian sleeping berry), 201
Witten-Herdecke University, Institute for Applied
  Epistemology and Medical Methodology, 22
World Health Organization (WHO), 5, 96

xylitol (sugar alcohol), 113–14

yarrow
  acid–base balance benefits, 203
  for detoxification, 181
Yawger, N. S., 105
yin and yang principle, 209

Zadeh, Lofti, 6
"Zahme Xenien" (Goethe), 29
ZC (zeolite clinoptilolite), 184–85
Zeitschrift für ärztliche Fortbildung (German
  Journal for Continuous Medical Education), 22
Zen Buddhism, 102, 103–4
zeolite clinoptilolite (ZC), 184–85
zinc
  acid–base balance benefits, 203
  immune system benefits, 68–69
  supplementation with, 186
zonulin, for testing leaky gut syndrome, 96, 184

About the Author

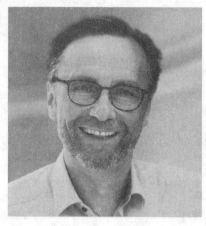

Mila Gligorić-Šmigić

Dr. Henning Saupe completed his medical studies at the University of Ulm, Germany, earning his license to practice medicine in Germany in 1992 and in Sweden in 1996. After completing his doctorate in the field of psychotherapy, he was also awarded the title of Doctor of Medicine in 1995. Dr. Saupe worked in Stockholm for ten years as a general practitioner with a focus on naturopathy, anthroposophical medicine, and holistic cancer therapy, and from 1997 to 2006, he served as a board member in the Swedish Association of Anthroposophic Physicians (LAOM). In January 2005, Dr. Saupe founded the Arkadiakliniken in Stockholm, the first hyperthermia clinic in Sweden specializing in oncological hyperthermia. He founded the Arcadia practice in Kassel in 2006 and in Bad Emstal, where he currently serves as medical director, in 2014. See www.arcadia-praxisklinik.de.

Since 2005, Dr. Saupe has regularly lectured in Scandinavia, including in Stockholm, Oslo, Gothenburg, and Malmö, as well as in the United States. In September 2007, he was awarded the Professor Olof Lindal´s Prize for Complementary Medicine at the Riksdag (House of Parliament) in Stockholm for his pioneering contributions of medical hyperthermia to complementary medicine in Sweden. Dr. Saupe is also a member of the ICHS (International Clinical Hyperthermia Society) and the DGO (German Society for Oncology). The father of three sons, Dr. Saupe lives in Bad Emstal, near Kassel, Germany.

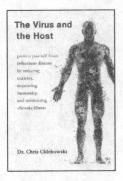
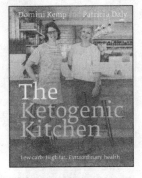
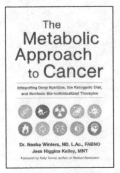
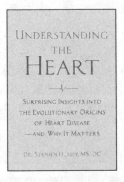
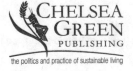

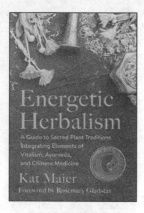
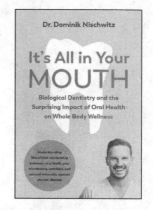
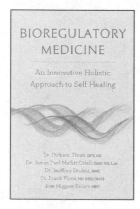
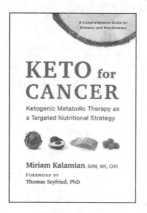
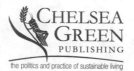